TWO MEALS A DAY

COOKBOOK

TWO MEALS A DAY

COOKBOOK

OVER 100 RECIPES TO LOSE WEIGHT & FEEL GREAT WITHOUT HUNGER OR CRAVINGS

MARK SISSON

with Brad Kearns and Sarah Steffens

balance

Balance
Hachette Book Group
1290 Avenue of the Americas
New York, NY 10104
grandcentralpublishing.com
twitter.com/grandcentralpub

First Edition: June 2022

Balance is an imprint of Grand Central Publishing. The Balance name and logo are trademarks of Hachette Book Group, Inc.

The publisher is not responsible for websites (or their content) that are not owned by the publisher.

The Hachette Speakers Bureau provides a wide range of authors for speaking events. To find out more, go to www.hachettespeakersbureau.com or call (866) 376–6591.

Print book interior design by Toni Tajima

Food photography © Natalie Kristeen Photography, based in Portland, Oregon. www.nataliekristeenphotography.com

Campfire illustration: Caroline De Vita
Chart design: Caroline De Vita

Special thanks to recipe consultant and chief tester Sarah Steffens (savorandfancy.com)

Library of Congress Control Number: 2022932826

ISBNs: 978-1-5387-3691-3 (paper over board); 978-1-5387-3692-0 (ebook)

Printed in the United States of America

WOR

33614082931113

10 9 8 7 6 5 4 3 2 1

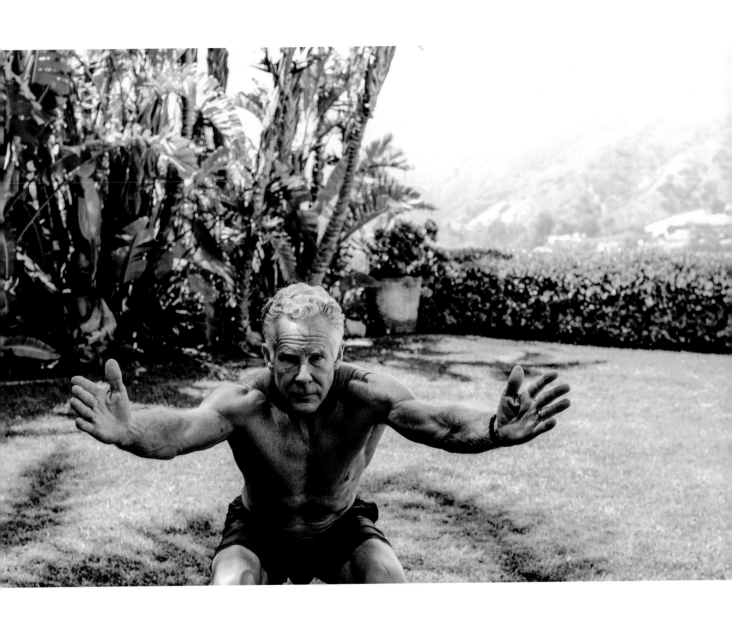

CONTENTS

PART I

INTRO-
DUCTION

THE

TWO
MEALS
A DAY

LIFESTYLE

CHAPTER 1

Thank you for your interest in this cookbook and in the passionate pursuit of healthful living! I am pleased to connect with you on the subject of eating delicious food. After all, it's one of the great pleasures of life, and it seems to be marginalized these days. The convenience of purchasing fast food to fuel a fast-paced lifestyle has become the cultural norm, and we have virtually forgotten the ancestral traditions of even the most recent generations. For those genuinely interested in eating nutritious, home-cooked meals, the controversy and confusion over what constitutes a healthy diet can be incredibly frustrating and discouraging. In *Two Meals a Day*, and this companion cookbook, I attempt to cut through all that noise and focus on a simple strategy that will maximize the nutrient density of your diet, help you efficiently drop excess body fat, and eat in a way that is enjoyable and sustainable forever.

Here's what is exciting about a *Two Meals a Day* lifestyle: it does not require the pain, suffering, and sacrifice that we have come to associate with restrictive diets and weight loss programs. Because you are ditching toxic modern foods and eating delicious meals that truly nourish your body at the cellular level, you always feel satisfied and naturally energetic, and maintain stable appetite, mood, and cognitive function all day long. This is true whether or not you eat regular meals! When you become an expert at burning body fat (and making ketones in the liver as needed), you will no longer be dependent on regular feedings of dietary carbohydrates as your primary source of energy. Carbohydrate dependency is a wholly modern affliction that drives all manner of disease and decline in modern life.

As you can learn from thousands of success stories published on my health information website, MarksDailyApple.com, losing weight and keeping it off is all about *hormone optimization*—escaping carbohydrate dependency and becoming what I like to call a fat-burning beast.

The idea that you can reach and maintain your ideal body composition while indulging in the lavish recipes contained in this book (and in many other ancestral-inspired cookbooks—see the Resources and Suggested Reading section), without worrying about portion control or painstakingly tracking macros, and without having to crush yourself working out, might seem too good to be true. But emerging science is validating that hormone optimization prevails over the traditional "starve and exercise" approach to fat reduction that has been a decades-long dismal failure. You see, when you try to lose fat by eating fewer calories and burning more calories, the body's compensatory homeostatic mechanisms will override your valiant efforts and push you back toward your so-called set point for body composition. After you pound the pedals at a 6 a.m. Peloton ride, you are triggered—both consciously and subconsciously—to consume more calories and burn less energy for the rest of the day. If you dutifully restrict portion sizes on a regimented diet, you'll become less energetic and

burn fewer calories, quickly adjusting to your new eating patterns without dropping any fat.

Over the long run, no amount of discipline or willpower can compete with these powerful hormonal and genetic drives. Recent books, such as Dr. Jason Fung's *The Obesity Code* and Dr. Herman Pontzer's *Burn*, have validated this concept, known as the *compensation theory*. Large-scale studies, like the Women's Health Initiative Dietary Modification Trial with fifty thousand women, have proven the folly of trying to bring about fat loss by calorie control. Subjects were predicted to lose thirty-two pounds of fat per year with diligent dietary modification, but after *seven years* of adhering to the program, the members of the group weighed virtually the same as when they started!

So, if pain, suffering, and sacrifice don't work, what are the real secrets to reducing excess body fat and keeping it off—and feeling healthy, happy, and energetic at the same time? Welcome to the *Two Meals a Day* lifeway! Although the essence of this eating strategy is to eat less frequently and choose the most nutritious foods, you cannot achieve a dietary transformation without adopting an assortment of complementary lifestyle factors, including fitness, sleep, and stress management. You see, hormone optimization and being a fat-burning beast are mostly about what you eat, but not entirely. A hectic, high-stress lifestyle of inadequate sleep, insufficient movement, poor fitness habits (exercising either too much or too little), or a flawed mindset can push you back in the direction of carbohydrate dependency and undisciplined eating habits.

Most of us have been deluded into believing that eating regular, grain-based, high-carbohydrate meals and snacks is aligned with health and vitality. You know, the all-American oatmeal and orange juice breakfast, a chicken sandwich with lettuce and tomato on wheat bread for lunch, low-fat energy bars in your snack drawer for a quick afternoon boost, and whole-grain pasta for dinner. Oh, and maybe some low-fat frozen yogurt for dessert. This menu doesn't sound too unhealthy in comparison to chomping French fries and guzzling soda, but we have to backpedal even further to unwind flawed programming and discover the truth about healthful eating. It is only since the advent of civilization around ten thousand years ago that humans have had ready access to high-carbohydrate foods. The hunter-gatherer lifestyle was a different story, and we were forced to become fat burners to adapt to the harsh "survival of the fittest" realities of primal life.

When we mainline processed carbohydrates and seed oils through most of our waking hours, we abuse the body's extremely delicate metabolic and hormonal functions that were designed to stabilize mood, energy, appetite, and cognitive function. Surprising as it may seem thanks to our deep immersion in carbohydrate-dependency dogma, humans can thrive without regular meals and snacks, and without today's wildly excessive carbohydrate intake in comparison to traditional *Homo sapiens* hunter-gatherer eating patterns.

Sugary beverages, snacks, and meals supply quick energy to the brain and muscles, but compared to fat, they are dirty-burning fuel sources. Fat, both from diet and from stores in the body, burns more cleanly through the utilization of mitochondria, the energy-producing power plants located inside most of your cells. When you consume lots of processed carbs (which are converted into glucose when ingested), you then produce lots of insulin to stabilize your blood glucose levels, which triggers system-wide inflammation and oxidative stress. These conditions are greatly exacerbated by the routine consumption of refined high polyunsaturated industrial seed oils like canola or soybean, which have toxic effects in the body and promote insulin resistance independent of excess carb intake. Oxidation and inflammation are widely regarded to be the root causes of all manner of disease, dysfunction, and accelerated aging. The high-carb intake, high-insulin production energy roller coaster is also perceived by your primal genes to be a stressful event with life-or-death consequences. Low blood sugar makes for an unproductive afternoon at the office but could have indeed spelled death during primal times.

Hence, your eating patterns prompt a chronic overstimulation of the delicate fight-or-flight response, leading to the disturbingly common modern affliction of burnout.

It's critical to make an immediate, all-out effort to escape carbohydrate dependency and develop the holy grail of health attributes that I call *metabolic flexibility*. This describes the ability to burn a variety of fuel sources to meet your precise energy needs at any given time, with the emphasis on stored body fat as your primary energy source. This approach to eating is aligned with our human genetic expectations for health—after all, it is our ability to gracefully burn fat (as well as store fat!) that drove 2.5 million years of human evolution.

To compare carb dependency with metabolic flexibility, it may be helpful to envision two different campfires. Carbohydrates burn like twigs and wadded-up newspaper. You get an instant big flame (sugar spike), with lots of smoke (free radicals generated by burning calories

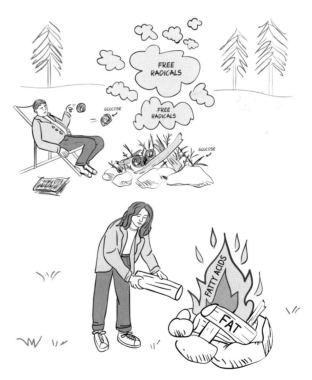

Glucose is like kindling on a campfire: it burns quick and dirty (free radicals) and needs frequent replenishment to keep the fire burning. In contrast, fat burns cleanly (mitochondria), like big logs supplying steady heat for a long time, and with no smoke.

without the protective benefits of mitochondria, as well as from the chronic overproduction of insulin). You have to constantly add more kindling (frequent meals and snacking) to sustain the fire. A fat- and ketone-burning beast has done the necessary work to make a beautiful campfire with big logs (stored body fat), glowing with warmth and burning cleanly (thanks to mitochondria) for hours without requiring much attention. This is why the fat burner enjoys peak physical and cognitive function even when skipping meals or significantly restricting carbs.

THE SISSON STANCE

At MarksDailyApple.com and on my social media accounts, my team and I field thousands of questions every week about all aspects of healthy living and the material I publish. The most common questions are along the lines of where I stand on dietary strategy and how to succeed with fat reduction. Whether it's politics, corporate brands, favorite sports teams, or dietary patterns, we often seek black and white answers to gain simple, on-the-go understanding from which to form fixed and rigid beliefs that we'll carry for a lifetime. When it comes to all aspects of healthy living, I think we can all benefit from taking a few steps back from this folly of black and white thinking to embrace a more mindful, nuanced, and thoughtful approach.

While the high-tech age allows us to exchange ideas and information more quickly and efficiently than at any other time in human history, we also face some novel challenges. Many healthy-living enthusiasts have plenty of awareness and knowledge of the basics, but as we further refine our approaches, things tend to get confusing, complicated, and overwhelming. Heck, athletics, fitness, diet, and nutritional science have been my obsession and avocation for decades, and I frequently feel confused and overwhelmed!

Although millions trust me as a health expert and ancestral movement leader, I've made a firm commitment to avoid forming or communicating fixed and rigid beliefs regarding health. Instead, I strive to maintain an open mind at all times, think critically, and dig as deeply as possible to get the real story from the most respected and scientifically validated resources. When presented with compelling science and anecdotal data or both, I have no problem revising some of my long-standing positions and recommendations. Indeed, I've rarely if ever been criticized for being wishy-washy or for flip-flopping; rather, I regularly receive appreciation for being flexible instead of heavy-handed. We're all doing the best we can on our collective journey toward optimal health, and we must never forget that personal preference and the overarching goal of enjoying life must surpass dogma every time.

Some recent examples of my evolution in dietary philosophy came with the emergence of the ketogenic diet around 2017, and the carnivore diet in 2019. I extensively studied the findings of keto research pioneers like Dr. Dom D'Agostino and Dr. Peter Attia, and wrote one of the first comprehensive books on the subject, *The Keto Reset Diet* (2017). However, as keto quickly exploded in popularity, I maintained a healthy distance from the hype and misappropriation of the science that emerged and continues to this day in the form of ridiculous weight loss pills and keto crash diets—all done in pursuit of instant results. I contend that keto is a fantastic tool to help heal from metabolic damage caused by decades of eating a high-carbohydrate diet, but it's not necessary to adhere to the strict ketogenic macronutrient guidelines over the long term.

While many experts initially dismissed, and continue to dismiss, the carnivore diet as an extreme and potentially dangerous fringe practice, I became increasingly intrigued by the

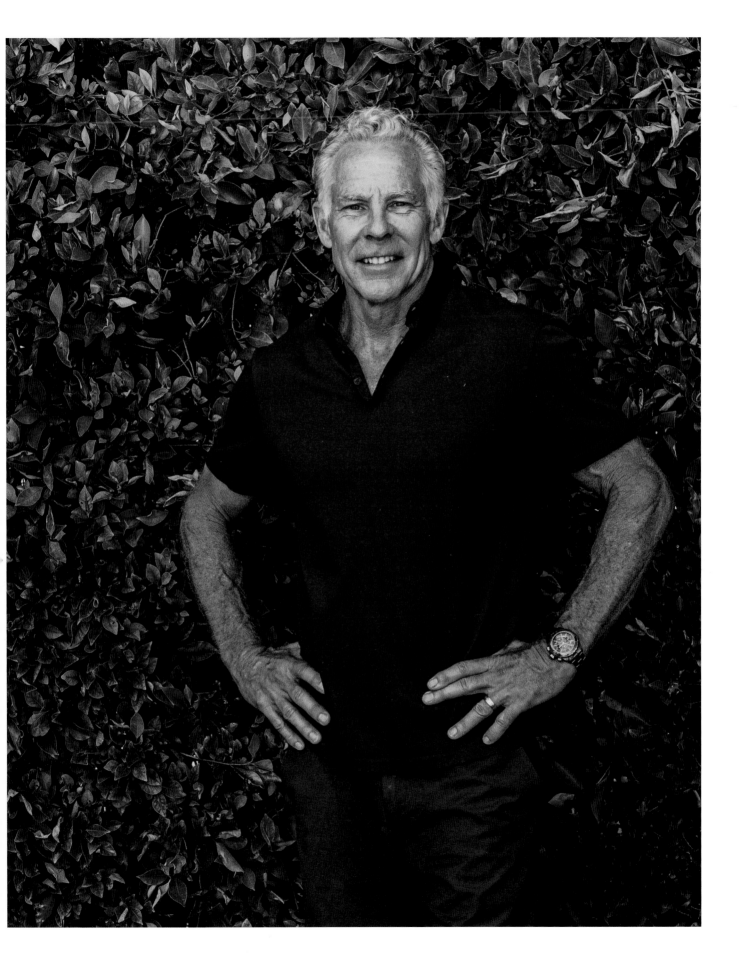

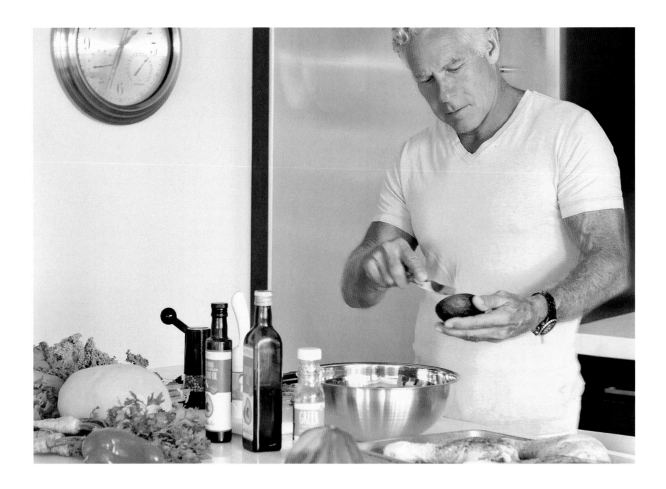

compelling message from movement leaders like Dr. Paul Saladino and Dr. Shawn Baker. Dr. Saladino, a board-certified psychiatrist, functional medicine practitioner, and author of *The Carnivore Code*, explains that plants contain natural toxins, or antigens, that they manufacture to ward off predators such as garden pests. For many, consuming plant toxins comes with an assortment of undesirable side effects. These include common digestion and elimination issues such as gas, bloating, flatulence, and diarrhea, but extend to all manner of autoimmune and inflammatory issues throughout the body. Gluten sensitivities and peanut allergies are some of the most prominent examples of plant reactivity, but adverse reactions happening at a subclinical level can add up to chronic inflammation when plants are consumed routinely. Unfortunately, we have been socialized to believe that plant consumption is obligatory for health, and that common adverse reactions are normal and perhaps a fair price to pay in exchange for nutritional benefits. It may be useful to consider the flatulence from eating beans or the bloated abdomen after drinking a super-nutrition green smoothie in a different light—as not normal or necessary but as adverse side effects from consuming these foods.

The carnivore argument compelled me to make some experimental modifications to my own longtime eating patterns, including challenging my fixed belief that vegetables are an essential dietary centerpiece. There is mounting evidence that an animal-based eating strategy can prompt incredible health transformations in longtime autoimmune and inflammatory condition sufferers, improve dietary nutrient density, and be an effective method of dropping excess body fat. The starting point with carnivore-style eating is to restrict consumption of all plant foods for at least thirty days and look for improvement with nagging health conditions, boosts in energy, focus, and mood, or success with fat reduction. Over time, you can experiment with adding the plant foods that have the least toxins, like raw honey, avocados, fresh berries, and sweet potatoes. Those with minimal sensitivities can add more plant foods as desired, always monitoring for any adverse reactions.

With the emphasis on nutrient-dense animal foods—such as sustainable land animals, oily cold-water fish, pastured eggs, the "nose-to-tail" cuisine such as organ meats and bone broth that is sorely lacking in the modern diet—along with the elimination of often problematic foods in the grain, legume, leafy green, and cruciferous vegetable categories, carnivore enthusiasts report improvements in assorted conditions, including the "leaky gut syndrome" that is being increasingly recognized as the root cause of many health problems. The rationale here is that meat and most other animal foods have few if any allergenic or toxin concerns for most people. In contrast, virtually all plant foods contain natural toxins that individuals may be sensitive to. This is why we have to soak, sprout, ferment, or cook most plant foods to render them edible. Some carnivore enthusiasts, like bestselling author Dr. Jordan Peterson and his daughter Mikhaila, thrive on a strict meat-only diet. Others can succeed with a carnivore-ish pattern in which the least toxic plant foods are integrated into the program. At the very least, if you have nagging conditions in the digestive tract or elsewhere, a thirty-day plant restriction experiment is warranted. Visit MeatRx.com to read hundreds of success stories attributed to the carnivore diet.

If you balk at the concept of restricting the colorful bounty from the plant kingdom in the name of health, note that progressive health enthusiasts are gaining a greater understanding and appreciation for the cutting-edge concept that there are *redundant pathways* to achieve the antioxidant and phytonutrient benefits provided by plants. *Hormesis* is the term for a brief, natural stressor (aka hormetic stressor) that delivers a net positive adaptive benefit. For example, fasting starves your cells of energy, prompting reactions such as making new mitochondria. Redundant pathways mean there are many ways to get an antioxidant boost besides drinking a freshly squeezed vegetable and fruit smoothie (and the accompanying megadose of sugar and plant toxins). The same antioxidant pathways that are activated by ingesting colorful berries (plant hormesis) are also activated by a cold plunge, a sauna session, or a period of fasting. The latter are examples of environmental hormesis.

My lifelong adherence to a high-carbohydrate, grain-based diet definitely came with some disastrous side effects that I was unaware of for decades. As an elite athlete obsessed with peak performance, I always chose the supposed best whole grains like brown rice and whole-wheat bread. I pounded organic nonfat yogurt, skim milk, and low-fat frozen yogurt, and snacked on the most natural and nutritious energy bars. Little did I know at the time, my devotion to conventional wisdom dietary recommendations was destroying my health. My extreme sensitivity to gluten and other natural plant toxins in assorted grains and legumes tore apart my digestive tract, resulting in chronic, systemwide inflammation and an assortment of autoimmune conditions. Fortunately, nothing was serious enough to require prescription drugs or hospital visits. However, I suffered silently and routinely with what has finally been validated by medical science as *leaky gut syndrome*. I endured persistent gas, bloating, and transient digestive pain for so long that feeling this way came to represent my "normal." My digestive sensitivities combined with the impact trauma of running 100 miles a week gave me leaky pipes to the extent that I literally had to design my running routes around restroom locations. I suffered from osteoarthritis in my feet and severe tendonitis in my hips, and experienced six or more upper respiratory tract infections a year. The aforementioned gastrointestinal maladies became severe when I was under periods of extra stress to the extent that they greatly compromised my enjoyment of life.

I'm sure glad I had an open mind to the novel and widely disparaged concept of the Paleolithic diet when it first emerged around the year 2000. When I cut all grains and seed oils out of my diet, I experienced immediate relief from decades-long suffering. This ranged from the front-and-center digestive issues all the way to corrections in weird conditions like arthritis in my hands when I played golf. Some twenty years into my ancestral health journey, I can honestly say I feel healthier and more energetic in my late sixties than when I was a world-class marathoner and triathlete in my twenties. While I have never detected any sensitivity to the toxins present in leafy greens or cruciferous vegetables, I have made a significant shift into what might be characterized as an animal-based diet with a sensible, but not essential, inclusion of plants. In plain speak, I've traded my legendary midday Sisson Bigass Salad for a midday Bigass Steak. This is mostly in the name of improving dietary nutrient density and avoiding possible subclinical plant sensitivities, as well as acknowledging that our need to consume plants for antioxidant benefits can be replaced via my sauna, sprinting, and cold plunging habits.

Another tenet I adhere to is to always honor the big picture of developing and honing metabolic flexibility through eating nutrient-dense foods, ditching junk food, doing intense workouts, increasing everyday movement, and prioritizing sleep. Certainly, we can add specific, well-executed dietary strategies like primal, Paleo, keto, or carnivore to this list, as well as precise protocols for fasting and compressed eating windows. After all, anything that introduces restriction and selectivity into the free-for-all of readily available processed foods is a positive! I also believe it's okay to stray from the narrow path now and then to have fun and enjoy life. For example, my extended family gathers for vacation at a different foreign venue each summer. Part of the fun is dining out together and exploring the unique offerings of local cuisine. I assure you that there are no continuous glucose monitors or

ketone blood strips happening on these trips, and I consume all kinds of fun foods that I would never integrate into my day-to-day dietary choices.

Hopefully, my story of ongoing dietary evolution will convince you to avoid drifting into rigid patterns, dogma, or a high-stress attitude toward eating. Instead, strive to maintain an open mind and a willingness to continually experiment and refine your optimal eating strategy. Remember, with the *Two Meals a Day* lifeway, you have the flexibility to honor your taste preferences, optimize your diet for special fitness goals, and change course if you experience health disturbances that you suspect are related to certain foods and food groups. Perhaps most importantly, it's imperative to avoid such a tightly wound approach to eating that the process becomes stressful. The term *orthorexia* refers to an unhealthy fixation on eating correctly, and it has become a significant concern among serious health enthusiasts. While it's critical to establish firm commitments and distinct boundaries with your food choices in today's processed food world, don't drift overboard into rigidity, obsession, or perfection.

I'm continually amused at the reaction I get from readers when I volunteer that I occasionally enjoy a slice of fresh baked bread dipped in cold-pressed olive oil and balsamic vinegar at a fine restaurant, add a pinch of sugar to my morning coffee, or enjoy homemade chocolate mousse or cheesecake at a birthday celebration. I have to reiterate that metabolic flexibility pertains not only to being skilled at fasting and burning stored body fat, but also to enjoying an occasional indulgence gracefully, then getting back to basics the next day.

On that note, make it count when you decide to indulge by choosing the absolute highest-quality products and appreciating the experience completely—no guilt or negative self-talk allowed! Choose a chemical-free, dry-farmed wine (visit DryFarmWines.com for details) when you want to imbibe. Source artisanal, bean-to-bar, Fair Trade dark chocolate instead of mass-produced brands that support child labor (check Askinosie

.com for an award-winning chocolate maker that shares profits with its equatorial farmers). By all means enjoy that hot apple pie fresh out of the oven when visiting Grandma. An occasional indulgence is significantly different from keeping your home environment stocked with nutrient-deficient, processed junk foods and consuming them mindlessly after an exhausting day. While I allow for little indulges here and there, I also have a firm policy of never eating anything that I don't absolutely enjoy. If there are no outstanding options available, as often happens when traveling, I take the opportunity to hone my metabolic flexibility through fasting. If you ever feel overwhelmed about all the nuances and sophistication of reaching ever-higher levels of healthful shopping, cooking, and eating, rest assured that most of your benefits will come from simply eradicating the Big Three toxic modern foods (more on this in the next chapter). Stay focused, stay positive, get right back on track after departures, and don't stress about it.

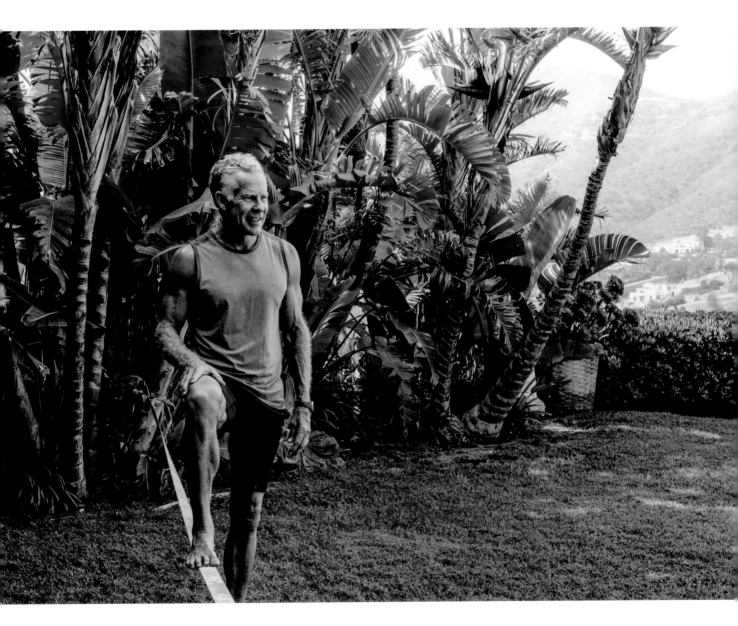

NINE TENETS TO SUCCEED WITH

TWO MEALS A DAY

CHAPTER 2

I encourage you to read *Two Meals a Day* for a comprehensive presentation on all aspects of healthful eating and complementary lifestyle practices, but I believe you can get the essence of this way of life by carefully reviewing and "owning" the following nine compelling tenets from the book.

1. DITCH THE "BIG THREE" TOXIC MODERN FOODS

The most important and urgent dietary modification is to eliminate what I call the Big Three toxic modern foods: *refined sugars, grains, and industrial seed oils*. You will find these offensive ingredients in most packaged, processed, and frozen foods in the supermarket, and in most convenience store and fast-food offerings. You can experience an amazing health transformation by eliminating these foods, which promote insulin resistance, inhibit the burning of body fat, and encourage carbohydrate dependency. Cleaning up your diet is the mandatory first step to escaping the epidemic disease patterns of obesity, metabolic syndrome, and type 2 diabetes. Don't pass Go and don't bother with any other details until you clean up your diet.

You've probably been exposed to plenty of information about the destructive effects of sugar and grains, but refined high polyunsaturated industrial seed oils, aka vegetable oils, deserve special scrutiny and disciplined elimination. Seed oils are extracted from the raw materials of corn, cottonseed, safflower, soybean, sunflower, and rapeseed (from which canola oil is derived). Unlike naturally oily olives, avocados, and coconut, which easily yield healthful and temperature-stable oils for cooking and eating, seeds don't easily yield oil. So, seed oils must be extracted using harsh chemical solvents and high-temperature processing methods. This results in oxidative damage to the product, damage that is greatly exacerbated when the oil is heated for cooking or used in making assorted baked, processed, packaged, or frozen food products.

These toxic agents are present in a variety of modern foods, particularly the bottled cooking oils that we were urged to switch to decades ago by flawed science and marketing propaganda inaccurately vilifying saturated fats. You'll also find seed oils prevalent in restaurant meals—not just fast food but also entrees cooked in these inexpensive oils at not only mid-level but also fine restaurants. Scrutinize labels and you'll find seed oils in all manner of packaged, frozen, and processed meals—from specialty ice creams to nearly all commercial salad dressings.

Seed oils are ingested and integrated into healthy fat cells, where they inflict immediate damage at the DNA level. Dr. Cate Shanahan, widely regarded as a leading crusader against seed oils, and author of *Deep Nutrition, Food Rules*, and *The Fatburn Fix*, explains that the level of destruction caused by these free radical–laden agents makes them "literally no different than eating radiation." Consuming these processed oils, aka Franken fats, on a regular basis inhibits your ability to burn stored body fat. For this reason, Shanahan and other experts contend that seed oils are the leading cause of insulin resistance, even more so than the high carbohydrate consumption that drives excess insulin production. Refined grains and sugars are objectionable as well, but as bestselling author of *Boundless*, extreme endurance athlete, and biohacking king Ben Greenfield explains, "With sugar, at least you can burn those calories off through hard exercise. Not so with industrial seed oils." When these toxic oils interfere with your ability to burn stored body fat, your system is compelled to obtain energy from dietary carbohydrates. Resolve to immediately eliminate these oils and all the nasty processed food that's made with them from your diet.

Immediately purge from your fridge and pantry the following offensive foods and food categories, and avoid consuming them when dining out:

- **INDUSTRIAL SEED OILS:** Bottled cooking oils (canola, cottonseed, corn, soybean, safflower, sunflower, and anything identified as "vegetable oil" or "vegetable shortening"); condiments with those oils listed on their labels (includes most mayonnaise, salad dressing, sauces, and dips, unless proudly stated otherwise on the label); margarines, buttery spreads, and sprays (Smart Balance, Promise, I Can't Believe It's Not Butter); deep-fried fast food; packaged and frozen baked goods; and most restaurant meals (ask them to cook your entree in butter instead of oil!).

- **SWEETS AND TREATS:** Bakery and pastry shop fare, candy and candy bars, cake, cheesecake, cookies, cupcakes, doughnuts, frozen desserts (ice cream bars, ice pops, and others), frozen yogurt, ice cream, milk chocolate, and pie.

- **SWEETENERS:** All artificial sweeteners (NutraSweet, Sweet'N Low, Splenda, and others), agave products, brown sugar, cane sugar, evaporated cane juice, fructose, high-fructose corn syrup, honey, molasses, powdered sugar, raw sugar, table sugar, and all syrups.

- **SWEETENED BEVERAGES:** Designer coffees (mochas, blended iced-coffee drinks); energy drinks (Red Bull, Rockstar, Monster Energy); bottled, fresh-squeezed, and refrigerated juices (acai, apple, grape, orange, pomegranate, Naked Juice, Odwalla, Nantucket Nectars, Ocean Spray, V8); overly sweetened kombucha drinks (read the labels—some are low in sugar, but most are not); sweetened almond, oat, rice, soy, and other nondairy milks (look for unsweetened); powdered drink mixes (chai-flavored, coffee-flavored, hot chocolate, lemonade, iced tea); soft drinks and diet soft drinks; tonic water; sports performance drinks (Gatorade, Powerade, Vitaminwater); sweet cocktails (daiquiri, eggnog, margarita); sugary cocktail mixes; and sweetened teas (AriZona, Honest Tea, Pure Leaf, Snapple).

- **GRAINS:** Cereal, corn, pasta, rice, and wheat; bread and flour products (baguettes, crackers, croissants, Danishes, doughnuts, graham crackers, muffins, pizza, pretzels, rolls, saltines, tortillas, Triscuit, Wheat Thins); breakfast foods (Cream of Wheat, French toast, granola, grits, oatmeal, pancakes, waffles); chips (corn, potato, tortilla); cooking grains (amaranth, barley, bulgur, couscous, millet, rye); and puffed snacks (Cheetos, Goldfish, Pirate's Booty, popcorn, rice cakes).

- **BAKING INGREDIENTS:** Cornmeal, cornstarch, and corn syrup; evaporated milk and condensed milk; flours made with wheat; gluten; starch; and yeast.

- **CONDIMENTS:** Review labels of condiments, sauces, spreads, and toppings. Discard those that contain sweeteners and seed oils and choose alternative products in categories such as ketchup, mayonnaise, salad dressing, and barbecue sauce (my Primal Kitchen products are made with an avocado oil base and are free from offensive ingredients); avoid all jams, jellies, and preserves (even all-fruit, no-sugar-added offerings).

- **DAIRY PRODUCTS:** Processed (American) cheese and cheese spreads (Velveeta); ice cream; nonfat and low-fat milks and yogurts; all other low-fat, high-carbohydrate dairy products; all nonorganic dairy products.

- **FAST FOODS:** Burgers, chicken sandwiches, fish fillets, french fries, hot dogs, onion rings, chimichangas, chalupas, churros, all deep-fried foods, and most everything offered at traditional fast-food establishments across the developed world. *Note:* Numerous modern fast-food chains offer much better choices than what's available at the typical burger joint. Chipotle and other "fresh Mex" offerings are good examples.

- **LOW-QUALITY FOODS ON THE ANCESTRAL LIST (SEE BELOW):** Conventionally raised meat and poultry from feedlot operations (choose grass-fed beef, pasture-raised fowl, heritage breed pork, and wild-caught fish instead—details in the next section); packaged meat products, such as smoked, cured, and nitrate-treated bacon; bologna, ham, hot dogs, gas-station jerky laden with preservatives, pepperoni, salami, and sausage (search for less-processed options in these categories, free from nitrates and other chemicals and preservatives); nonorganic eggs, milk, and other dairy products (choose those that come from pasture-raised animals and are sustainably harvested, or at least certified organic); nonorganic produce with a high pesticide risk (those with difficult-to-wash or edible skins, such as leafy greens and berries); produce out of season or transported from distant origins (fresh local summer berries, thumbs-up; big-box-store pineapples and mangoes in wintertime, thumbs-down); nuts, seeds, and nut butters processed with oils or covered in sugary coatings; most farmed fish and imported fish (especially farmed Atlantic salmon).

2. EMPHASIZE ANCESTRAL FOODS

Humans evolved to digest an incredible variety of colorful, wholesome, nutrient-dense plants, animals, and even insects. While there are genetic variations that influence whether you struggle or thrive on certain foods, we are incredibly resilient when it comes to obtaining the nutrition and the caloric energy we need from what's available in our environment. While I strongly support personal preference as the driving force in your dietary choices, we must always honor our human genetic expectations for health and choose from the natural plant and animal foods that fueled human evolution for 2.5 million years: meat, fish, fowl, eggs, vegetables, fruits, nuts, and seeds. You can add certain healthful modern foods to your options, including organic high-fat dairy products and high cacao percentage dark chocolate. From this broad list, you can certainly exclude foods you don't enjoy and emphasize foods and meals that you have discovered through trial and error to work well for you. Here is how to choose wisely in each category:

Meat and Fowl

All the objections to eating meat can be mitigated by sourcing local, sustainable, grass-fed, or certified organic meat whenever possible.

In contrast, mass-produced feedlot animals are raised in objectionable environmental and health conditions, and given hormones, pesticides, and antibiotics to prevent illness and increase yield in crowded, unsanitary, polluting environments.

The ideal choice is a local animal that was 100 percent grass-fed or pasture-raised. Get familiar with your nearby farmers' markets, natural-foods grocers, and food co-ops. Explore specialty butchers and international markets for variation beyond the mainstays (cow, pig, chicken, turkey), such as lamb, buffalo or bison, and venison. These animals were more likely to be grass-fed and sustainably harvested. If your local options are limited, there are many great internet resources, including ButcherBox.com, ThriveMarket.com, USWellnessMeats.com, and WildIdeaBuffalo.com. (See Resources for more.)

Fish

Fish and other marine life have been a centerpiece of the human diet for millennia and rank among the most nutrient-dense foods on earth. Seafood is a fantastic source of omega-3 fatty acids (especially the hard-to-find DHA and EPA types) and contains a broad spectrum of vitamins, minerals, and antioxidants. Oily, cold-water "SMASH" fish (sardines, mackerel, anchovies, wild-caught salmon, and herring) have the highest omega-3 values and overall health benefits and are quite affordable. The shellfish family (clams, crab, crayfish, lobster, mussels, oysters, shrimp, scallops) is also highly regarded for its unique and potent nutritional offerings. The high zinc content in oysters boosts testosterone and dopamine, giving them a well-deserved reputation as an aphrodisiac. The widely popular canned tuna is nutritious and affordable; look for environmentally sensible brands. Be sure to expand your consumption of seafood to include the nutritional superstar seaweed—namely, kombu, kelp, nori, and wakame.

As with conventionally raised meat, selectivity is warranted with fish consumption. Avoid all packaged, processed, boxed, or frozen dinner preparations, especially breaded and deep-fried offerings. In general, strive to avoid most types of farmed fish, especially the predominantly farmed Atlantic salmon—it's typically raised in cramped conditions with harmful food additives. Pass on fish imported from the Baltic Sea, Chile, and Asia because of concerns about polluted waters, chemical use, and long transport times. Avoid predatory fish (king mackerel, mahi-mahi, marlin, shark, swordfish, big tuna) because of their potentially high levels of mercury and other contaminants. Avoid fish that are endangered or caught by environmentally damaging methods (visit MontereyBayAquarium.org for details).

Eggs

Eggs are the original superfood—the essence of life—and deliver across-the-board nutritional benefits. Egg whites contain high-quality complete protein, while the yolks are a treasure trove of antioxidants, anti-inflammatory compounds, healthful omega-3 and saturated fats, and vitamins A, E, K_2, B complex, and folate. Eggs are particularly high in choline, which boosts memory and cognition and supports cell maintenance and DNA synthesis.

Local, farm-fresh eggs sold by hobbyists or farmers' market vendors are the premier choice, as these chickens enjoy an active and omnivorous outdoor lifestyle. Their diet of insects, lizards, worms, weeds, grasses, and seeds yields eggs with vastly superior nutrient density to those of feedlot chickens. Notice the vibrant orange yolks and rich taste for confirmation of higher omega-3 and other nutrients than in the dull yellow, watery yolks from feedlot chickens. Beyond a true local farm-fresh egg, strive to purchase cartons labeled "pasture-raised" and "certified humane" or "animal welfare approved." USDA certified organic eggs are the next best option. Pastured eggs and organic eggs are in widespread distribution, so strive to avoid conventional eggs or those with unofficial designations like "natural diet," "free-range," or the like. Consider trying alternative eggs like duck, quail, or other animals outside the industrial food system.

Vegetables

Vegetables have high levels of antioxidants, flavonoids, carotenoids, and phytonutrients that help optimize metabolic, immune, and cellular functioning. They help protect the brain and the body from the ravages of aging and oxidative stress and help nourish healthful bacteria in your gut microbiome. Vegetables grown above ground (leafy greens, peppers, asparagus, tomatoes) and those in the cruciferous family (broccoli, cauliflower) are high in complex carbohydrates and low in starch, with abundant fiber and water content. Root vegetables (beets, carrots, onions, parsnips, rutabagas, sweet potatoes, turnips, yams) are grown in the ground, where they absorb high levels of antioxidants, vitamins, and iron from the soil, making them nutritional powerhouses. Their high starch content makes them a great choice for reloading glycogen after strenuous exercise. Root vegetables, along with fruits, are among the least toxic plant foods, making them a good choice for carnivore-style eaters looking to safely include plants and carbs in their meals. Avoid white varieties of potatoes, because they are starchier, highly glycemic, laden with pesticides, and less nutritious than potatoes with colored flesh.

Prioritize local, in-season, pesticide-free vegetables from farmers' markets or natural-foods grocers. USDA certified organic is the next best choice. Insist on organic produce for vegetables with a large edible surface area (spinach, kale, leafy greens) or those whose skin is consumed, or difficult to wash (bell peppers, celery, cucumbers). Avoid vegetable juices, which are too concentrated in sugar. If you believe you may have sensitivity to the natural toxins contained in plants, evidenced by frequent gas, bloating, and digestive pain and chronic autoimmune or inflammatory conditions or both, avoid raw vegetables and consider further restrictions in pursuit of healing.

Fruit

Fruit is a great source of broad-spectrum antioxidants and micronutrients, but some selectivity is warranted if you are trying to shed excess body fat. Prioritize locally grown, pesticide-free, in-season fresh fruits. Berries, avocados, lemons, limes, and stone fruits (cherries, peaches, apricots) are the top choices, as they have the highest antioxidant values and the lowest glycemic values. On the flip side, strive to avoid eating fruit in the wintertime, avoid high-sugar dried fruits and dates, and try to de-emphasize the high-glycemic tropical fruits such as banana, mango, papaya, and pineapple.

Nuts, Seeds, and Their Derivative Butters

Nuts and seeds are nutritional powerhouses rich in protein, fatty acids, enzymes, antioxidants, phytonutrients, and abundant vitamins and minerals. Numerous large-scale dietary studies suggest that regular consumption of nuts, seeds, and their derivative butters significantly reduces the risk of heart disease, diabetes, and other health problems. These foods are extremely

satiating and have been touted as an excellent snack option that will help ease the early stages of transition from carbohydrate dependency to metabolic flexibility. On the other hand, nuts and seeds are among the more problematic for food sensitivity and intolerance, and some complain that their caloric density can interfere with fat-reduction goals.

Be sure to find packaged nut options that are raw or dry-roasted, because many leading brands contain refined industrial seed oils that are used during processing. Read labels carefully! Consume fresh nuts within six months or store them in the freezer to extend shelf life. If the nuts you have on hand start to smell oily or rancid, or if they develop flecks on their surface, discard them. Don't worry about obtaining organic nuts, because the protective shell negates pesticide concerns. Nut butters are gaining in popularity. If you can find the rare but decadent delicacies macadamia nut butter or coconut butter (Brad's Macadamia Masterpiece has both, at BradVentures.com), they rank right up there with dark chocolate as a delicious, satisfying treat to replace your old sugary options. Single-serving nut butter packets are great for convenient energy on the go and are a perfect replacement for high-sugar sport gels.

High-Fat Dairy Products

Choose raw, fermented, unpasteurized, unsweetened, high-fat, low-carbohydrate, organic selections—including ghee and butter; full-fat cream, cottage cheese, and cream cheese; and raw or certified organic whole milk—from pasture-raised and grass-fed animals. You can also enjoy organic fermented dairy products, including cultured buttermilk, full-fat Greek yogurt, kefir, raw-milk cheese and aged cheese, and full-fat sour cream. Avoid all low-fat and nonfat milks, yogurts, cottage cheese, imitation dairy products (whipped cream, creamers), and frozen treats. Strive to consume only organic dairy products, because conventional dairy is laden with hormones, pesticides, and antibiotics. Even the routine homogenization and pasteurization of dairy products can cause digestive disturbances and reduce nutritional benefits. Dairy is a highly allergenic food category, so if you detect adverse inflammatory or autoimmune reactions, be sure to stick with raw, organic, high-fat, or fermented options.

Dark Chocolate

Dark chocolate is a delicious and nutritious treat with numerous health benefits and a low carbohydrate content. High cacao, bean-to-bar dark chocolate is one of the richest dietary sources of antioxidants (polyphenols, flavanols, catechins) and is teeming with phytonutrients and broad-spectrum minerals, including iron, chromium, copper, magnesium, and manganese. Dark chocolate also contains a powerful opioid peptide called *phenylethylamine*, aka the love drug. This hormone-like substance acts as an amplifier for numerous mood-elevating neurotransmitters such as dopamine, serotonin, and norepinephrine. Dark chocolate is the most prominent dietary source of an agent called *theobromine*, which has cardiovascular benefits; acts as a natural stimulant, appetite suppressant, and memory booster; and reduces inflammation. *Epicatechin* is another prominent flavonoid in dark chocolate that has been found to boost nitric oxide production, which improves arterial function.

Dark chocolate is labeled according to the percentage of ingredients, by weight, obtained from the cacao bean. A 100 percent cacao bar has no added sugar and a bitter taste. A milk chocolate or semisweet chocolate bar has tons of sugar and milk powder added, putting it in an entirely different food category than dark chocolate—that is, a sugar bomb! Strive to consume bars that are at least 70 percent cacao and acclimate over time to bars that are 85 percent or higher. Select only premium, handcrafted, artisan bars—look for designations such as "bean-to-bar," "single origin," and "Fair Trade" on the label, and always be sure the first ingredient is cacao beans. Expect to pay at least triple the price for a quality bar ($3 to $5 per ounce) versus mainstream, mass-produced bars at the typical retail price point of around $1 per ounce. Understand that these major brand bars are made with bulk ingredients of unknown origin, including substandard, over-roasted cacao beans. In addition, if you choose mainstream, lower-priced bars, you can be certain you are supporting child labor in poorly regulated African cacao-producing countries.

Seek out great internet resources and establish direct relationships with artisan bean-to-bar chocolate makers who support fair wages and working conditions for their sourcing farmers. Askinosie.com is an award-winning American chocolate maker that shares profits with their equatorial farmers. CocoaRunners.com and BarAndCocoa.com offer a vast selection of bean-to-bar chocolates from around the world. Become a chocolate connoisseur and enjoy one square at a time on your tongue—do not bite into a bar! Store in a cool, dry place, but never refrigerate.

Animal Organs

The ancestral tradition of consuming the entire animal in a nose-to-tail manner has been tragically left behind in our modern cuisine. Although we consume high-quality, sustainable muscle meats such as steak, hamburger, and chicken breast, we neglect the most nutritious parts of the animal. You can easily find and enjoy budget-friendly animal superfoods such as liver, heart, kidney, and other organ meats (known as offal), bone-in cuts of meat, and authentic gelatinous bone broth. These foods have been a centerpiece of traditional diets around the globe for thousands of years and for eons of hunter-gatherers before that.

You can start your superfood mission with liver, arguably the most nutrient-dense food on the planet (oysters and salmon roe could compete here, too). Liver has outstanding levels of B vitamins, iron, zinc, magnesium, phosphorus, selenium, folic acid, choline, and fat-soluble vitamins (A, D, E, and K). For example, beef liver has seventeen times more B_{12} than ground beef. Liver is the only meaningful dietary source of retinol, the fully formed state of vitamin A that delivers comprehensive anti-inflammatory benefits. If you have trouble with liver's strong taste, consider making a puree of liver and grass-fed hamburger and frying up some superfood burgers, or consuming raw, frozen, salted chunks of liver. Experiment with other organs such as brain, heart, kidney, oxtail (tailbone), Rocky Mountain oysters (testicles), tripe (stomach lining), tongue, and sweetbread (thymus or pancreas). Tania Teschke's *The Bordeaux Kitchen* integrates organs into numerous interesting and tasty French cuisine recipes.

Bone broth and bone-in cuts of meat are the best dietary sources of the important but hard to find nutrients collagen and glycosaminoglycans. These agents support hair, skin, nail, and connective tissue health and are believed to have a "heal and seal" effect on your all-important gut lining. Choose an authentic bone broth brand that lists bones as the first ingredient, specifies a long cooking time on the label, and turns gelatinous when refrigerated. Don't confuse real bone broth with the prevalent watery version found in cartons that are labeled chicken, vegetable, or beef "broth." These will remain liquid even when refrigerated and do not have the nutrient density of real, gelatinous broth. For your organ meats, find a quality butcher or natural-foods grocer in your area, or an internet resource such as USWellnessMeats .com. It's critical to find grass-fed organ meats, because organs contain more fat than muscles, and any toxins present tend to concentrate in fat cells. Organ meats are ridiculously affordable because they are still unpopular.

Fermented and Sprouted Foods

Fermented and sprouted foods are some of the best sources of probiotics, which nourish healthful intestinal bacteria and lay the foundation for excellent digestive, immune, hormonal, and cognitive functioning. Suggestions include apple cider vinegar, raw or aged cheese, kefir, kimchi, kombucha, raw milk, miso, natto, olives, pickles, sauerkraut, tempeh, and full-fat yogurt. These foods contain live cultures ready to nourish your healthful gut bacteria. Some fermented foods, including wine, beer, sourdough bread, and cacao, don't contain live-culture probiotics but still offer a variety of health benefits.

3. REMEMBER THAT *WHEN* YOU EAT IS JUST AS IMPORTANT AS *WHAT* YOU EAT

Today's epidemic rates of insulin resistance (the inability of cells to properly respond to the signaling of insulin), type 2 diabetes, obesity, cancer, heart disease, and all other diet-related disease and dysfunction are driven by eating too much of the wrong foods, too often. We've all heard plenty of commentary about the hazards of junk food and the wonders of nutritious food, but not enough attention is paid to eating frequency. When we eat and snack throughout our waking hours, even when taking care to consume nutritious foods, we can still inhibit fat burning and fat loss, promote system-wide inflammation, overproduce insulin, and dysregulate important hormonal functions. Of course, we need calories to fuel our bodies for busy days and ambitious workouts, but we have forgotten our magnificent, genetically hardwired ability to store, manufacture, and burn various forms of energy to enjoy active, productive lifestyles. *Homo sapiens* possess what I like to call "closed-loop functionality": we can maintain steady energy and alertness all day long, regardless of the type of calories we ingest or how frequently we ingest them. These mechanisms evolved by necessity to help us survive the rigors of primal life, when there was no guarantee of a "next meal."

Amid today's obsession with fad diets, exotic juice cleanses, wonder supplements, and regimented eating strategies, it's important to realize that the human body operates most efficiently in a fasted state. Fasting allows us to access ancient pathways of cellular renewal and regeneration, where immune function, cognitive function, cell repair, and antioxidant and anti-inflammatory processes are all optimized. The simple act of skipping a meal beats any exotic antioxidant, fresh-squeezed juice, or superfood preparation for an immediate health boost, hands down. This insight should feel like a relief to those immersed in health and wellness. I believe it takes the pressure off to realize that not only is your body going to be okay if you miss your morning green plant juice blend or afternoon energy bar, but it will be better in every way.

When it comes to dropping excess body fat and preventing diet-related disease, you can focus on ditching processed foods and eating less frequently. While snacking on nutritious foods may be necessary at the outset of your journey to help you make the sometimes difficult transition from carbohydrate dependency to fat adaptation, realize that even a healthful snack will immediately halt the burning of stored body fat and prompt an insulin response. The idea with *Two Meals a Day* is to naturally and gracefully progress from whatever your starting point is—without any pain, struggle, sacrifice, or deprivation—to enjoying a *maximum* of two nutritious meals a day with little or no snacking. While my typical daily pattern involves a midday steak for lunch and an evening restaurant meal, there are many days where I'll have only one major meal, paired with an extended fast or a mini meal at another time of day. This strategy is especially effective when traveling, as I believe fasting during the journey and then immediately syncing your meals to your new time zone is a fantastic strategy to beat jet lag.

Besides a natural optimization in caloric intake that comes from eating a maximum of two main meals with little or no snacking, there are other benefits to eating less frequently. Emerging research on the concept of time-restricted feeding (particularly from Dr. Satchin Panda at the Salk Institute for Biological Studies in San Diego, Dr. Valter Longo at the University of Southern California, and Dr. Jason Fung, author of *The Obesity Code*) suggests that our bodies are highly attuned to a digestive circadian rhythm that is strongly aligned with our overall sleep-wake circadian rhythm cycles. Our digestive system needs downtime from eating and processing calories, and this is particularly true after dark.

Resolve to strictly limit your digestive function to a maximum of twelve hours per day and strive to minimize eating after dark. Granted, this is tougher to do in the winter than the summer, but make your best effort. As you progress with your metabolic flexibility, see if you can compress your eating window from a twelve-hour baseline. Many enthusiasts favor a 16:8 strategy, where the typical daily fasting period is sixteen hours, and all calories and meals are consumed within an eight-hour window (e.g., noon to 8 p.m.). Eating less frequently and getting competent at fasting is the gateway to metabolic flexibility, dropping excess body fat, and minimizing your disease risk factors.

4. DO IT THE RIGHT WAY

The comprehensive health benefits and fat loss potential of fasting and eating two meals a day are possible only when you are able to burn stored body fat effectively. If you try to jump into aggressive fasting or carb restriction efforts without first establishing the ability to burn stored body fat, you are going to struggle royally, trigger a prolonged fight-or-flight reaction, and eventually experience the backsliding and burnout that are so common with ill-advised crash diets. Hence, it's essential to proceed step-by-step toward metabolic flexibility; adopt a comprehensive lifestyle approach with attention to fitness, sleep, and stress management; and never take on any challenges that make you feel fatigued, frustrated, or discouraged.

Of course, processed foods are the biggest driver of insulin resistance and type 2 diabetes, but poor sleep habits, insufficient daily movement, lack of high-intensity exercise, and too much general stress in everyday life are all major contributors to metabolic dysfunction and disease patterns. You can think of it this way: stress, fatigue, and burnout drive carb consumption, while an active, fit, stress-balanced lifestyle with plenty of rest and recovery promotes fat burning. This rule is independent from your food choices! The most glaring example here is the widespread propensity toward overtraining among devoted fitness enthusiasts in endeavors like CrossFit, endurance running and triathlon, and hard-core boot camp, spin class, and Peloton participants. Engaging in a pattern of exhausting, depleting workouts promotes strong cravings for carbohydrates. This can happen immediately after the workout, and it can happen when your 6 a.m. spin class pairs reliably with a 9 p.m. pint of ice cream. Only by reducing exhausting workout patterns does one have a fighting chance at staying aligned with ambitious dietary transformation goals.

Granted, when you clean up your act by eating fewer calories and minimizing or eliminating processed foods, you'll probably feel great for a little while. After all, any departure from a junk food lifestyle is going to be a net positive. However, if high-carbohydrate meals and snacks have been your primary energy source for decades and you suddenly decide to convert into a keto machine or fasting ascetic, you are likely to trigger the prominent fight-or-flight mechanism of *gluconeogenesis* to supply your immediate energy needs. This is the catabolic process of converting lean muscle tissue into glucose for instant energy as part of the body's emergency response. You may have experienced this when you faced a sustained personal crisis like an intense work deadline or family hospital vigil, when you felt alert and energized even when you didn't take the time or have the appetite for healthy meals. Alas, the fight-or-flight response is designed for immediate and emergency use only; think about our ancestors needing to persevere with hunting and gathering efforts despite facing starvation. Sure enough, after a few weeks or a few months, your emergency fueling systems will eventually become exhausted and you will arrive at the familiar modern destination of burnout.

You can avoid the pitfalls of crash dieting by pursuing the vaunted health attribute of metabolic flexibility in a natural, graceful, and sustainable manner. It starts with cleaning up your diet while you also optimize the various lifestyle factors that can make or break your dietary success. Take comfort knowing that the *Two Meals a Day* journey should feel comfortable and easy to maintain at all times. Struggling with energy level swings or appetite spikes indicates that your approach needs fine-tuning, or that you are trying to progress too quickly. Often, adding some additional carbs, eating plenty of nutrient-dense, ancestral-style foods, correcting erratic training or sleeping patterns, and not trying to shed body fat until later will help you quickly correct course and keep the momentum going.

A safe and effective way to hone skills of fasting and metabolic flexibility is to simply wait until WHEN (when hunger ensues naturally) to eat your break-fast meal every day. This takes the pressure off having to reach arbitrary mealtime goals, such as the more advanced 16:8 strategy. Even more importantly, the WHEN strategy will reestablish your long-lost hunger and satiety signals, which have been compromised by overeating and the regimented meal patterns that have become cultural norms.

5. GET YOUR MIND RIGHT

It's easy to get frustrated, confused, and discouraged when pursuing diet and fitness goals with the typical "struggle and suffer" approach. It's time to eliminate and reframe self-limiting beliefs, forgive yourself for past failures, and form an empowering new mindset that you deserve exceptional health and the body you dream of. Believing this deeply (and reaffirming it regularly through journaling, positive affirmations, and making healthy choices) will help you stay focused and leverage small successes into long-term habits.

The first step in getting your mind right is to acquire the self-knowledge of what it takes to succeed. This entails having a firm understanding of what foods and eating strategies are truly healthful and effective, and rejecting assorted flawed and dated conventional wisdom relating to diet. For example, headline stories about red meat causing cancer have contributed to its bad reputation, but looking further into the research it's easy to reject this distorted and misinterpreted message. Studies disparaging red meat typically group all types of red meat together (ignoring how grass-fed steak is an entirely different food from heavily processed bologna or a chemical-laden fast-food hamburger), fail to account for the influence of consuming unhealthy refined carbs and seed oils in conjunction with red meat, and also rely on questionable data. Errors in data can range from inaccurate self-reporting of dietary habits from the study population to failing to account for confounding variables such as adverse lifestyle practices that exacerbate diet-related disease.

Armed with a clear conviction of how to eat healthfully, next you must understand any strengths, weaknesses, and blind spots that can potentially interfere with your success. For example, if you tend to stay up late enjoying electronic entertainment, you may discover that this pattern is connected with reaching for sugary treats at night.

Harboring a negative self-image is one of the most common areas of struggle. Failure is so commonplace with diet, fitness, and body composition goals that it's easy to attach your self-esteem to your repeated failures and subconsciously give up before you even start. It can be valuable to start doing some gratitude journaling or meditation exercises at the outset of pursuing a daunting goal. Whatever your current state of health, eating patterns, and body composition, you can cultivate some level of compassion for your past mistakes and shortcomings, and gratitude for possessing a decent starting point (it could always be worse!), acknowledging that you have boundless potential for improvement.

With an open heart and a clear head, you can embark upon dietary and lifestyle transformation. Strive to appreciate the process and not become overly fixated on results. The changes will come naturally when you feed and care for your body at the highest possible standards of health. If you notice old destructive thoughts and behavior patterns creeping into the picture, you can gently take control of your thoughts and emotions instead of panicking and backsliding. It's all about redirecting negative thoughts into thoughts of self-compassion, self-acceptance, and gratitude.

Get into a rhythm where healthful meal choices and lifestyle practices can feel natural, sustainable, and enjoyable. It's very difficult if not impossible to harness the flimsy motivator of willpower to be at your best every day. Psychology experts contend that willpower is a diminishing resource. If you have to constantly restrain yourself from eating the wrong foods or rally theatrically to get your tail out the door for some exercise, your willpower and motivation can eventually weaken to the extent that you succumb to the constant temptations of comfort, convenience, and instant gratification. You may choose eating a treat instead of brushing your teeth and heading to bed, or settle in for video entertainment instead of a workout or a walk.

Set yourself up for success by establishing firm rules and guidelines that align with your goals and do everything you possibly can to create a winning environment. For example, make the commitment to start your day with some sort of movement routine that you can make into a habit (e.g., walk the dog around the block, perform a sequence of yoga sun salutation poses, or tackle a more elaborate session such as "Brad Kearns Morning Routine" on YouTube). Establish a rule that you will complete your movement routine before reaching for your phone and getting sucked into the vortex of nonstop electronic stimulation and distraction that is part and parcel of the digital age. Purge from your home all offensive foods, and don't allow them to enter your shopping cart or creep back into the picture over time. Someday you may find yourself staring at a slice of birthday cake during a celebration, but this is a vastly different scenario from habitually buying and consuming nutrient-deficient foods. Spend some time doing advance preparation so that you always have healthy meal options available; this will help reduce the likelihood that you will reach for processed foods in a pinch. To encourage movement breaks and regular exercise, create easy opportunities in your home and work environment. For example, place a kettlebell in plain view so you can do a few swings at any time. Install a pull-up bar in a doorway and hang resistance cords from the bar so they are ready at a moment's notice. When fitness opportunities are within your visual field all day long, there is much more likelihood that you'll take advantage of them than if your fitness equipment gets relegated to a corner in the basement or a closet.

We need repetition and endurance to form winning new habits and allow flawed beliefs and behavior patterns to fade into the background and eventually vanish forever. Take some time to write down positive affirmations and post them in a prominent spot for everyday viewing. Set alarms on your devices to remind you to get up and take regular movement breaks. Write down a simple sequence of exercises constituting a micro-workout and post it right next to the pull-up bar and resistance cords.

Consider going deeper into the brain reprogramming realm to create a vision board or a mind movie. A vision board is a visual representation of your dream life, complete with aspirational photos of cars, homes, vacation destinations, impressive physiques, and inspirational quotes. A mind movie, promoted by law of attraction expert and bestselling author Joe Dispenza, entails creating a homemade video filled with imagery of life goals and dream scenarios, inspirational music, and positive affirmations. You then watch the movie repeatedly to elicit positive thoughts, emotions, and behaviors. Learn about the morning "priming" exercise recommended by peak performance guru Tony Robbins; it involves breathing, visualization, gratitude, and relaxation exercises to reprogram the subconscious mind toward "love, passion, and success."

Hey, I realize this stuff takes time and energy and is off the beaten path of your hectic daily schedule and never-ending to-do list. It's easy to form a skeptical mindset that such exercises are silly or futile. If this is the belief that you hold, you are most certainly correct! On the other hand, if you agree to cultivate an open mind and make a healthy effort in some of these ideas, you may just experience great things happening in your life.

6. FOLLOW A FAT-BURNING LIFESTYLE

Healthy eating is only one piece of the big picture. Complementary lifestyle habits can make or break your efforts toward dietary transformation. We have a critical need not only to optimize evening sleep, but to constantly balance stressful daily life with sufficient recovery and downtime. The most urgent objective is to minimize artificial light and electronic stimulation after dark. Cultivate calm, dark, mellow evenings so you can transition gracefully into a good night's sleep. It's also important to discipline your use of technology to achieve regular downtime from hyperconnectivity. This will allow your brain to refresh and refocus on peak cognitive tasks and renew your appreciation for live social interaction and the simple pleasures of life, such as appreciating nature.

Evening Sleep

A good night's sleep allows your brain and body to repair and rejuvenate from a stressful modern life. It's the centerpiece of a healthful lifestyle from which all other healthful lifestyle practices emanate. It's not worth attempting dietary transformation or tackling an ambitious fitness regimen until you get your sleep dialed in. Unfortunately, modern life is all about excess artificial light and electronic blue light exposure after dark. This violently disrupts our all-important circadian rhythms and the extremely delicate hormonal functions that for millions of years have been calibrated to the rising and setting of the sun.

The simple correction here is to make your evenings more mellow and relaxing. Strive to end your screen use at least an hour, and ideally two hours, before bed. Implement calming bedtime rituals, such as a final stroll around the block with the dog (wear light clothing to lower body temperature; this is a great trigger for sleep), quiet reading or conversation, or a

warm bath. Minimize the lighting in your home, using UV-blocking lenses, orange light bulbs, and candlelight instead of bright indoor lighting. A good night's sleep actually starts first thing in the morning: strive to awaken naturally, near sunrise, and immediately get outdoors for some direct exposure to natural light. Interestingly, emerging research cited by Dr. Andrew Huberman, Stanford University neuroscience professor and host of the *Huberman Lab* podcast, suggests that getting adequate exposure to natural ultraviolet light during the day has an appetite-suppressing effect.

Recovery and Downtime

Our natural opportunities for downtime and cognitive refreshment have been obliterated by mobile technology, extended (or endless) remote workdays, and the efficiencies that make life "easier" in many ways, but often more hectic and jam-packed. We have an urgent imperative to create opportunities for rest, rejuvenation, and downtime like no other period in the history of humanity.

It takes tremendous discipline and focus to power down from hyperconnectivity and reprioritize live social interactions, solo reflective time, and passive existence in natural surroundings, so you must establish rules, guidelines, incentives, and alternative activities to minimize the temptation of hyperconnectivity. Eating can be a great catalyst here. Make an effort to prepare delicious home-cooked meals from scratch and include friends and loved ones for a grand social experience. Establish strict off-hours for your mobile device and email availability. Make an effort to spend time in nature. While the most intense natural surroundings provide the maximum benefit (ocean swimming, mountain hiking), relaxing in your backyard or local park can also bring emotional, spiritual, and cognitive rejuvenation. Japanese research on "forest bathing" reveals that even brief connections with nature can lower stress hormones and prompt a strong parasympathetic response.

When you fall behind in life, napping is a great strategy to quickly refresh brain neurons and help you feel alert, energized, and renewed in as little as twenty minutes. When it comes to exercise, it's important to emphasize recovery in your training program, and steer clear of workouts and workout patterns that are overly stressful and can lead to breakdown, burnout, illness, and injury.

7. INCREASE GENERAL EVERYDAY MOVEMENT

Increasing all forms of general everyday movement, especially taking breaks from prolonged periods of stillness, is now deemed more important to health than following a devoted workout regimen. Calories burned during workouts don't contribute to fat loss as we've long believed (due to the constraints on daily calorie burning and compensatory mechanisms discussed earlier), but moving throughout the day prompts the genetic signaling for fat burning and appetite regulation. Walking should be the central focus of your movement activity, and you can also engage in dynamic stretching, calisthenics, brief bursts of explosive exercise, and formal movement practices such as yoga, Pilates, and tai chi.

Walking is the quintessential form of human locomotion but seems to be a lost art in modern life. Granted, countries like Australia and Switzerland set a stellar example with citizens achieving the widely cited goal of ten thousand steps per day (about 5 miles) and a strong cultural and infrastructural focus on walking. In contrast, Americans accumulate only around half that in average daily step count, which earns us the official designation as a sedentary population.

Today, it's necessary to orchestrate opportunities to walk and engage in other movement practices instead of succumbing to the comforts, conveniences, and indulgences that tempt us around every corner. It's especially important to avoid prolonged periods of stillness, which can hamper fat burning and cognitive function in real time and increase disease risk over the long term. Try some fun countercultural strategies such as routinely parking at the far edge of the parking lot instead of trolling for the closest possible space to the store. Resolve to take stairs instead of elevators from this point forward for the rest of your life. No excuses! If you need to get to the twenty-seventh floor, get off at the twentieth and finish on the stairs. Stop at the park during your commute home and take a leisurely lap or two before you transition into relaxation mode at home. If you own a dog, answer to a calling higher than yourself and give the animal the life it deserves. Through mud, rain, sleet, snow, or whether you feel like it or not, get the dog out three or four times a day for a quick stroll and a longer outing. The morning exercise routine mentioned earlier makes a great contribution to your daily movement quota and helps with overall habit forming for an active lifestyle.

To be clear, I don't want you to feel intimidated by another to-do list item of taking long walks or other prolonged cardio sessions to meet a movement quota. A few minutes here and there add up to huge benefits, especially as it relates to getting up from stints at your desk or on the couch. Similarly, while a yoga class can be a blissfully immersive mind and body experience, doing short pose sequences here and there on days when you're pressed for time can augment your formal classes. If you are an enthusiast of traditional cardio activities such as jogging, running, cycling, triathlon, and the like, be sure to exercise at a comfortable, completely aerobic pace, keeping your heart rate at or below "180 minus your age" in beats per minute.

8. CONDUCT BRIEF, EXPLOSIVE WORKOUTS

Traditional fitness programming tends toward excessive and overly stressful steady-state cardio exercise, or the popular but often exhausting high-intensity interval training (HIIT) protocol. Research is conclusive that challenging your body with occasional brief, explosive, all-out efforts of resistance exercises or sprints delivers phenomenal fitness benefits. This is the missing link for many devoted fitness enthusiasts! Some experts, like *Body by Science* author Dr. Doug McGuff and *P:E Diet* coauthor Dr. Ted Naiman, contend that just *minutes* of properly conducted explosive exercise can deliver superior fitness benefits compared to hours of lower-intensity workouts.

The trick is to challenge your body with maximum efforts that elicit temporary muscular failure. This will prompt your profound genetic signaling to come back stronger, faster, leaner, and more resilient. While there are numerous benefits to leading an active lifestyle featuring assorted forms of exercise, you will get vastly more return on your investment when you go hard once in a while. Unfortunately, the majority of fitness enthusiasts never tap into their high-intensity performance potential because they either stick to steady-state cardio or conduct high-intensity workouts incorrectly. It's essential to limit your all-out efforts to less than ten seconds so you can achieve maximum force production throughout the sprint down the track or during a set of aggressive kettlebell swings. Then, take extensive recovery time between efforts—at least a 6:1 rest-to-work ratio (sixty seconds of rest after ten seconds of work). Explosive effort with extended rest will enable you to repeat a similar high-quality performance and minimize the cumulative fatigue that can occur when you repeat too many work efforts with insufficient rest between. As you progress through reps, if you notice your performance deteriorating even slightly, it's time to end the workout. Remember, the goal is to prompt an optimal hormonal response and genetic signaling, not to become exhausted and depleted.

An ideal sprint workout for anyone from novice to experienced athlete would be an extensive warmup, dynamic stretching, preparatory technique drills, and a primary set of sprints lasting around ten seconds each, with at least sixty seconds of recovery between these short sprints. Depending on your fitness level, complete from four to ten reps, then cool down and call it a day. You should feel pleasantly fatigued at the end of the session, but certainly not fried, exhausted, and craving sugar. A little goes a long way with explosive exercise, so performing several short resistance workouts (under thirty minutes) and a single sprint workout each week as described is plenty.

While adding explosive workouts is critical to your success, you must also take extra care to avoid overtaxing yourself during these sessions. Monitor your energy levels at rest to avoid crash-and-burn patterns where you can't stay awake in the afternoon following a morning sprint session. If you experience recurring muscle soreness after tough sessions, dial everything back a few notches so you don't have to routinely allocate extra resources to repairing muscle damage. As you include the explosive stuff, also introduce specially designed workouts that promote recovery through low-intensity cardio, dynamic stretching, mobility and balance drills, breathing exercises, and foam rolling.

9. PURSUE BIG BREAKTHROUGHS!

After you have done the hard work to ditch the Big Three toxic modern foods, emphasize nutrient-dense ancestral foods, and adopt the complementary lifestyle behaviors of excellent sleep, frequent movement, high-intensity workouts, and rest and recovery, you are poised to pursue ambitious body composition and performance goals. Advanced techniques can be very effective when you want to take those often-difficult incremental gains from good to great. To drop excess body fat and keep it off, you need to shock your body with occasional stressors that are brief and deliver a net adaptive benefit.

Following are some ways to signal your genes to shed excess body fat relatively quickly. Once you reach your body composition goal, you should be able to maintain your new physique indefinitely without much trouble. Even if you back off from these advanced strategies, reduce the amount you exercise, and get a little loose with your diet, or all of the above, your homeostatic drives and compensatory processes will help keep your body-fat percentage within a tight range.

Extended Fasting

This is an excellent weapon that can be unleashed on a regular basis to make swift progress toward your body composition goals. After building up sufficient momentum with the WHEN strategy, hopefully it will be no trouble to adhere to a 16:8 pattern on most days of the week. From there, you can throw in the occasional challenge day where you try to extend fasting beyond the sixteen-hour mark to spur a boost in metabolic flexibility. Strive to reach the esteemed standard of a twenty-four-hour fast now and then, as this will put you in the highest category of metabolic flexibility. While advanced enthusiasts promote strategies like OMAD (one meal a day!), occasional seventy-two-hour fasts, or even five-day fasts, a "more is better" mentality is not necessary here. Excessive or overly stressful fasting can trigger adverse metabolic and hormonal consequences in certain individuals, especially active, athletic females who already have low body fat or those who are ill prepared for such challenges.

An intuitive approach can be highly effective for extended fasting. There will be certain days where you don't feel like eating or don't have access to excellent food choices, so take these opportunities to conduct an extended fast. While the WHEN strategy requires that you eat upon experiencing hunger sensations, see if you can work through a hunger spike now and then. The prominent hunger hormone ghrelin, which gets your stomach "growlin'" with the secretion of digestive enzymes, spikes for around twenty minutes to compel you to eat. After that period of time, if your body realizes it's not getting food any time soon, the ghrelin spike will subside and you will start to accelerate fat burning and ketone production. You may be able to comfortably extend your fast for much longer than you think, until you reach a point when you'll really enjoy a nutrient-dense meal.

Fasted Workouts

Pairing fasting with intense or prolonged exercise starves your cells of energy and prompts the highly beneficial process of *mitochondrial biogenesis*—making additional energy-producing mitochondria in your cells. You can play around with numerous variables to determine what works best for you, including the duration of your fast before exercise, the duration of your fast after exercise, and the duration and intensity level of your workouts. Be sure that the degree of difficulty of your efforts is appropriate. You should not feel weak, hungry, or fatigued during fasted workouts, nor drained and depleted afterward. If you experience an energy crash in the hours after a fasted workout or have difficulty recovering, dial back one or more variables the next time out.

One safe and sensible starting point is to fast overnight, conduct a challenging workout in the morning, and then replenish calories WHEN. From there, you can experiment with starting the workout later in the morning or perhaps waiting one to three hours after the session to consume calories. See if you can experience true sensations of hunger at some point after your session, then try to ride it out for twenty to sixty minutes before eating. Waiting out a hunger spike can effectively upregulate fat-burning genes, not only in the moment but for hours and days afterward. Remember, it's all about sending the right signals to your genes to be able to provide necessary energy for ambitious exercise, as well as stabilize mood, energy, and cognitive function for hours afterward even if no food is available.

It's extremely important to avoid overstressing yourself when you conduct fasted workouts. For long-duration aerobic sessions, your heart rate should always remain in the aerobic zone, which is calculated by subtracting your age from 180 and keeping your heart rate at that number or below in beats per minute. For high-intensity sessions, be sure that you maintain a *consistent quality of effort* throughout the workout. This means explosive output with impeccable technique for each work effort, extensive rest between work efforts, and ending the workout before cumulative fatigue, form breakdown, and cellular damage from overstress occur.

Sprinting

While some metabolic mechanisms are beyond direct scientific explanation, anecdotal data from the fitness and athletic world strongly confirm the insight that "nothing cuts you up like sprinting." You'll get the most benefit from high-impact sprinting on flat ground, but low- and no-impact sprints (stairs, hills, stationary bikes, rowing machines, and other cardio machines) are also excellent fat-burning catalysts. Sprinting sends a powerful genetic signal to shed excess body fat because the performance drawbacks from carrying excess body fat while sprinting, or jumping for that matter, are more severe than with any other athletic activity. It may be difficult to believe that a workout with only one to five minutes of maximum effort can generate profound health, fitness, and metabolic benefits, but it's the adaptive response in the hours and days afterward where the real magic happens. This is known as the *afterburn effect*, where your body works hard to return to homeostasis and responds to the organism being stressed to the maximum. These adaptive mechanisms include rebalancing hormone levels, replenishing glycogen, synthesizing protein, replenishing ATP, increasing fatty acid oxidation, improving oxygen delivery to the muscles, recruiting more explosive muscle fibers, and of course shedding unnecessary body fat.

The most important maxim to remember with sprinting is that a little goes a long way. Workouts that last too long, are beyond your current ability level, or are performed too frequently with insufficient rest between will not optimize the adaptive response. Instead, you will increase your risk of breakdown, burnout, illness, and injury. It's essential to put aside the "no pain, no gain" mentality and conduct workouts that are brief and always explosive, and that you can recover from reasonably well. Slight next-day muscle soreness and fatigue are expected, but if you feel trashed and super stiff after these sessions, sprint for a shorter duration, take more rest between efforts, or perform fewer reps.

As you grow fitter and stronger over time, focus on going faster rather than adding reps or shortening your recovery time. If you have to start your sprinting journey with low- or no-impact options, try to progress toward running high-impact sprints eventually. Running stairs or uphill sprints is a great progression workout, as you will build running competency with less impact trauma. Next, try to integrate some "wind sprints" into your workout. These are brief accelerations of around four seconds where you approach high speeds, then gradually decelerate for around four seconds. You can also perform an assortment of running technique drills that will both prepare you for sprinting and deliver an excellent high-intensity workout. Search YouTube for "Brad Kearns Running Technique Drills" for both basic and advanced lessons. Hopefully one day you will be blasting some maximum-effort sprints and enjoying the comprehensive health, fitness, and body composition benefits.

Therapeutic Cold Exposure

Anecdotal evidence and cutting-edge science are revealing the incredible potential of therapeutic cold exposure, aka cold thermogenesis, to stimulate fat reduction both independently and as a complement to diet and exercise efforts. Exposure to cold water is particularly therapeutic because its greater molecular density (versus air) drains body heat twenty-five times faster than exposure to cold air. Taking a cold shower—or, better yet, plunging into a tub or natural body of near-freezing water for a few minutes every morning—triggers an intense hormonal response. You experience an immediate and sharp increase in alertness and motivation as well as accelerated fat metabolism for hours afterward.

Exposure to cold not only prompts additional calorie burning as the body seeks to rewarm, it provides an opportunity to reconnect with our ancestral past and one of the key hormetic stressors to make us lean, strong, and resilient creatures. Evolutionary anthropologists believe that routine exposure to cold was a key evolutionary driver of optimal endocrine and immune function as well as efficient fat metabolism. Today, we exist primarily in temperature-controlled environments (research reveals that the average modern citizen spends 93 percent of life indoors!), and an assortment of human survival attributes have atrophied accordingly. By implementing a basic cold exposure practice, you can fine-tune fat metabolism, improve thermoregulatory mechanisms, and boost psychological resilience to not only cold, but all other forms of stress you face in everyday life.

Exposure to cold activates brown adipose tissue (BAT), a special kind of fat that is not routinely burned for energy but instead exists to keep us warm. When BAT (concentrated in the shoulders and upper back) is activated, it triggers an increase in the burning of regular stored body fat, also known as white fat. Besides brown fat activation, a cold plunge delivers a fantastic burst of energy, alertness, and euphoria. You are tapping into ancient adaptive processes and response mechanisms that are hardwired into our genes. One prominent Finnish study revealed that immersion into 40-degree-Fahrenheit water (4.4 degrees Celsius) for even as few as twenty seconds spikes the prominent mood, focusing, and motivation hormone norepinephrine by 200 to 300 percent for up to one hour! Cold exposure also delivers profound anti-inflammatory, immune-boosting effects, including an increase in the production of the internal super antioxidant glutathione. And cold exposure prompts the release of beneficial cold-shock proteins, which facilitate an assortment of repair processes in brain synapses and muscle tissue.

While brown fat activation is a reliable fat-burning booster, realize that cold exposure is believed to trigger an increase in appetite. The trick here is to endure an appropriate amount of cold, then try to rewarm naturally over the ensuing hours—perhaps paired with fasting. If you experience the predictable spike in appetite after your cold session, see if you can ride it out. Remember, a ghrelin spike will persist for around twenty minutes, then subside. While the research is still mixed on whether therapeutic cold exposure is a verifiable weight loss catalyst, Dr. Andrew Huberman offers plenty of validation for a so-called shiver protocol that boosts fat metabolism. Huberman recommends experiencing cold to the point of a mild shiver, getting out for a bit and allowing the shiver to resolve naturally, then re-entering the cold for a few cycles. Huberman explains that cycling in and out of the water is preferred to trying to extend the duration of your sessions, because any potential fat-burning boost is minimized when you acclimate to the cold over time. Shivering is the catalyst for accelerated fat burning, and it's not too daunting to induce a bit of a shiver before taking a break.

You can embark upon a cold therapy protocol by simply cranking the shower handle to full cold for the final one or two minutes of your shower and progressing at a comfortable pace to running a few cycles of cold for two minutes or as long as it takes to induce shivering. Hopefully, you will appreciate the exhilaration of cold exposure, the immediate mood boost, and the fat-burning benefits to become a serious enthusiast. Search YouTube for "Brad Kearns Chest Freezer Cold Water Therapy" for a primer on the ultimate home therapy protocol of immersing into a large, top-opening chest freezer filled with cold water.

LET'S EAT!

CHAPTER 3

I recommend you quickly skim through the recipes and mark those of most interest to you. Then you can plot out a strategy and start compiling a grocery list to get going with some delicious meals. You'll notice that macronutrient calculations are provided for each recipe. This will help you obtain a basic understanding of the calorie composition of certain food categories and meals, and assist you in hitting any daily protein goals for your body weight. Most experts recommend getting an average of around 0.7 gram of protein per pound (1.54 grams per kilo) of lean body mass (total body weight less body fat weight) daily. If you feel the need to carefully track your calories and macros, there are numerous websites and apps you can utilize. FitDay, MyFitnessPal, My Macros+, and Senza are a few popular resources.

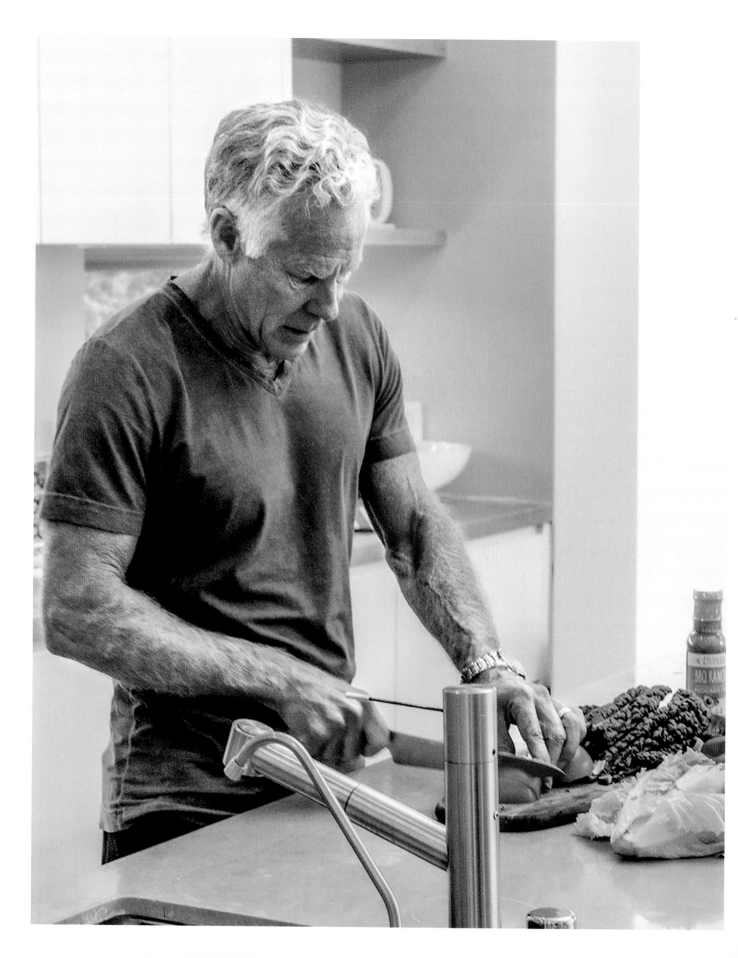

Here is an overview of the recipe categories:

BREAK-FAST AND EGG-BASED ENTREES: You'll see an emphasis on eggs, the traditional morning food, but these recipes are great to eat at any time of day. You can't beat pasture-raised eggs for superfood affordability and cooking convenience.

SAVORY APPETIZERS: Meatballs and more are great to have around when you want something substantial but don't have time to prepare a full, proper meal. These preparations will be the talk of the party potluck too!

CHICKEN, TURKEY, AND MEAT ENTREES: Fire up your grill, get your cast-iron skillet out, or use your pressure cooker for these tasty recipes featuring pasture-raised fowl, grass-fed beef, and heritage breed pork. These recipes range from simple preparations with minimal ingredients to more gourmet recipes for those special occasions when you have more time and energy. When you source the most sustainably raised meats, you boost nutritional value and minimize moral and environmental objections to eating meat.

ORGAN MEAT ENTREES: Organs were a centerpiece of the ancestral human diet and are widely regarded as the most nutrient-dense foods on earth. They remain a fixture in many traditional cuisines around the world but have been egregiously neglected in the fast-food era. These preparations will allow you to reconnect with your ancestral past and help you replenish depleted cellular energy with truly superfood meals.

CARNIVORE-ISH ENTREES: These recipes will boost the nutrient density of your diet, provide an incredible level of satiety, and also allow you to perform a plant food restriction experiment in hopes of improving nagging inflammatory or autoimmune conditions. A carnivore-ish strategy has also been shown to be effective for fat reduction. You will consume minimal carbohydrates but feel totally satisfied after each meal.

SEAFOOD ENTREES: Don't forget about all the wonderful nutrients and healthy fats found in fish and shellfish! Not only are these recipes delicious, but they are easy to make and don't require much time to prepare. You'll have more time to crush your goals and to-do list, so what are you waiting for?

VEGGIE-ISH ENTREES: I come in peace to spread love and good cheer to all healthy eating enthusiasts across the planet! While choosing to adhere to a vegan or vegetarian eating strategy is a high-risk endeavor because you will be avoiding the most nutrient-dense foods on the planet, you can certainly enjoy many meatless dishes as meals or sides.

SMOOTHIES: The modern smoothie is presented as an antioxidant powerhouse and energizer for healthy folks, but it's typically a sugar bomb. It can also be a plant toxin bomb when you throw in tons of raw leafy greens. This chapter will awaken you to new possibilities where natural, nutritious fats are the prominent calorie source, and you can conveniently add assorted superfoods and supplements in the blender (e.g., animal organ capsules, creatine, collagen, glutamine, magnesium, whey protein), without worrying about integrating all these nutrients into meal recipes.

DESSERTS AND TREATS: Granted, the Two Meals a Day program offers a strong recommendation to avoid snacking, but the desserts and treats category is in line with the "enjoy life" edict. If you are going to indulge, let's make sure you are avoiding cheap processed ingredients and can actually obtain some nutritional benefits along with sensational taste.

REALLY FAST, EASY MEALS FOR PEOPLE WHO ARE TOO BUSY TO COOK: This is my nomination for most clever category title! It also addresses my biggest pet peeve when I look at my shelf with dozens of outstanding cookbooks full of fabulous recipes. I've enjoyed some amazing one-off preparations, but I notice that if they require too many ingredients, too many steps, and too much time, they won't make it into my regular rotation. This section is dedicated to real people leading real lives—enjoy!

CARNIVORE SCORES FOOD RANKINGS

This chart from Brad Kearns and health coach Kate Ouellette-Cretsinger ranks the most nutrient-dense categories of animal-sourced foods and makes suggestions for strategic inclusion of numerous colorful, healthful plant foods that have the least toxicity and most nutritional benefits. If you are suffering from nagging autoimmune or inflammatory conditions, it's absolutely worth performing a thirty-day dietary restriction experiment in which you avoid plant foods and emphasize nose-to-tail animal foods. Monitor your symptoms carefully to assess improvements. Over time, you can strategically add back the least-offensive plant foods, as described in the chart. The carnivore-ish strategy is also effective for weight loss because it provides excellent nutrient density and highly satiating protein, and is low in carbohydrates.

The Carnivore Scores Food Rankings chart will keep you focused on the true superfoods of the planet, especially when some of these foods have been marginalized in modern commerce and culture. It will also help you navigate to the best choices in each food category. Strive to accept nothing less than the most sustainably raised animal products. Even if you're on a tight budget, realize that you can score well on the chart with extremely affordable options like liver and other organs, the SMASH fish family, and pastured eggs. You may be surprised at the "steak line," and the concept that red meat scores higher than chicken, turkey, and pork, but experts like Dr. Cate Shanahan confirm that their nutrient density is inferior to that of red meat, especially if the animals have been mass-produced. Notice the supplement options if you can't seem to get enough liver and bone broth into your meal plans.

K8 4 Wellness BRAD'S

CARNIVORE SCORES!

Follow this chart to eat smart; plants à la carte

 ANCESTRAL SUPPLEMENTS

MAXIMUM NUTRIENT DENSITY

GLOBAL ALL-STARS ▶ The world's most nutrient-dense foods (sorry kale, time to bail).	**Grass-fed Liver** *(Bonus points: consume raw or medium rare)* Superior micronutrient profile, including off-the-charts in vitamin A and vitamin B group.	**Oysters** *(Lightly grilled, broiled, or roasted, never deep-fried)* Aphrodisiac properties are validated by the incredible zinc and B$_{12}$ levels.	**Salmon Roe and Caviar** Rich in iodine, choline, omega-3 fatty acids EPA and DHA.
ANIMAL ORGANS ▶ Reclaim the forgotten ancestral tradition of "like supports like."		**Liver plus Bone Broth Heart, Kidney, Sweetbread, Rocky Mountain Oysters, Tripe** Choose grass-fed animals.	**Organ Supplements (Capsules)** AncestralSupplements.com: freeze-dried, 100% grass-fed organs (capsules) PrimalKitchen.com: collagen peptides (powder)
WILD-CAUGHT, OILY, COLD-WATER FISH ▶ Convenient, affordable, best dietary source of omega-3s.		**"SMASH" Family:** Sardines, Mackerel, Anchovies, Salmon, Herring	
SHELLFISH ▶ Excellent source of monounsaturated and omega-3 fats. Choose sustainably caught/raised.		**Oysters plus Clams, Crab, Lobster, Mussels, Octopus, Scallops** Sushi bar fare!	
EGGS ▶ Healthful fats, choline, B vitamins, and life-force essence.		**Local, Certified Humane and Pasture-Raised** Vastly superior to conventional.	**Other Eggs: Goose, Duck, Quail, Ostrich** Healthier animals; no mass production.
RED MEAT ▶ Superior nutritional and fatty acid profile to poultry.		**Local or 100% Grass-fed** Bone-in cuts best.	**Other Red Meat: Buffalo/Bison, Elk, Lamb, Venison** Healthier animals, no mass production.

THE STEAK LINE

Emphasize foods above line for maximum dietary nutrient density.

Chicken, Turkey, Pork Inferior nutrient density and fatty acid profile if corn/soy fed.		Local or 100% grass-fed/pasture-raised poultry; heritage breed pork		
Raw, Organic, High-Fat Dairy Avoid all conventional, pasteurized, and low- and nonfat products, or if allergic.		• Raw cheese (aged, hard, or Brie), raw kefir, raw milk • Cream cheese, heavy cream, sour cream • Full-fat yogurt		

Plant Foods Integrate strategically for recovery/glycogen reloading, to improve insulin sensitivity, optimize thyroid and adrenal function, and enjoy life!	**Avocados**	**Dark Chocolate**	**Fermented Foods**	**Fruit**
	Heart-healthy monounsaturated fats, huge potassium, high antioxidant, vitamin B$_6$ and vitamin K.	Super high in antioxidants, flavanols, polyphenols; choose bean-to-bar, 80 percent cacao or higher.	Kefir, kimchi, kombucha, miso, natto, olives, pickles, sauerkraut, tempeh; probiotics nourish healthy gut bacteria.	Choose locally grown, in-season fruits; berries #1 for low glycemic/high antioxidant properties.
	Honey	**Nuts & Nut Butters**	**Seaweed**	**Sweet Potatoes/Squash**
	Choose raw for antioxidant, antibacterial boost. Local honey can help seasonal allergies.	Nutritious protein, fatty acids, enzymes, antioxidants, phytonutrients, vitamins and minerals. (bradventures.com).	Best source of iodine, vitamin D, vitamin B$_{12}$, selenium, and omega-3.	High antioxidant, anti-inflammatory, immune-boosting and support gut health.

Check out BradKearns.com/MOFO and K84Wellness.com for more great info and guidance.

PART II

RECIPES

BREAK-FAST AND EGG-BASED RECIPES

CHAPTER 4

You'll see an emphasis on eggs, the traditional morning food, but these recipes are great to eat any time of day. You can't beat pasture-raised eggs for superfood affordability and cooking convenience. Enjoy!

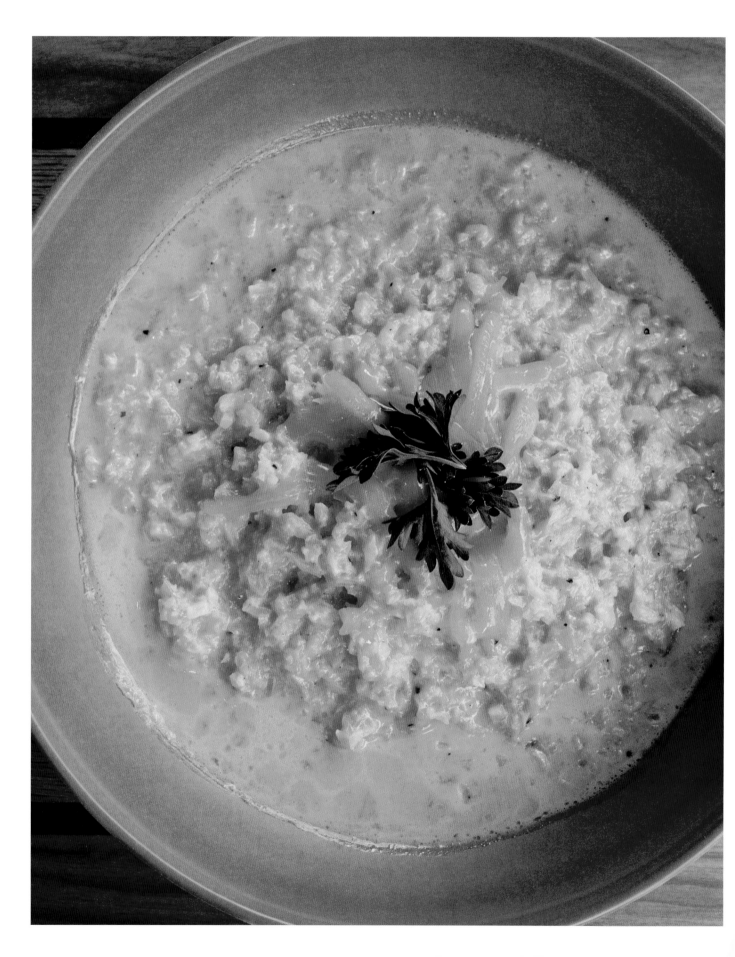

KETO BREAKFAST GRITS

This bowl of keto grits will satisfy your craving for a warm and creamy breakfast without spiking your blood sugar and robbing your energy. This is delicious as is, or you can top with minced bacon, seared shrimp, or wilted greens.

- 4 tablespoons (60 g) butter
- 4 cups (400 g) riced cauliflower
- 1 teaspoon (5 g) sea salt
- ½ teaspoon (1 g) black pepper
- 1 teaspoon (1.25 g) garlic powder
- 1 cup (240 mL) heavy whipping cream
- 2 cups (480 mL) plain and unsweetened almond milk
- 1 cup (114 g) shredded Cheddar cheese
- Fresh parsley, for garnish

INSTRUCTIONS:

Melt the butter in a Dutch oven or large soup pot over medium-low heat. Add the riced cauliflower and sauté until soft, about 5 minutes.

Season with sea salt, black pepper, and garlic powder and stir well to combine.

Stir in cream and almond milk, reduce the heat, and simmer until thickened, about 10 minutes.

Remove from the heat, stir in the shredded cheese, and serve. Store leftovers in an airtight container in the fridge for up to 5 days.

SERVES 4

PREP TIME: 5 MINUTES

COOKING TIME: 15 MINUTES

CALORIES: 526

CARBS: 11

PROTEIN: 9

FAT: 51

DENVER OMELET SALAD

If you are a fan of the Denver omelet, this hearty salad is right up your alley! You can increase the fats in this dish with a sprinkle of shredded cheese or some diced avocado.

SALAD:

- 8 cups (240 g) baby spinach
- 1 tablespoon (15 g) butter
- 4 large eggs
- 1 medium (150 g) yellow onion, sliced
- 3 garlic cloves, minced
- 1 teaspoon (5 g) sea salt
- ½ teaspoon (1 g) black pepper
- 1 medium (150 g) green or red bell pepper, seeded and diced
- 1 cup (140 g) cubed ham
- 1 cup (200 g) tomatoes, chopped

VINAIGRETTE:

- ½ cup (120 mL) extra-virgin olive oil
- ¼ cup (60 mL) raw apple cider vinegar
- 1 teaspoon (5 g) sea salt
- ½ teaspoon (1 g) black pepper

INSTRUCTIONS:

Arrange the spinach leaves on a platter.

Melt the butter in a skillet over medium heat. Crack the eggs into the skillet and fry, flipping once, until done to your liking. Transfer the eggs to a plate and set aside.

Add the onion, garlic, sea salt, and black pepper to the skillet and sauté until soft, about 5 minutes. Add the bell pepper and continue to sauté for another 5 minutes. Add the ham and sauté until the ham has heated through, 3–5 minutes.

Scoop out the veggie and ham mixture and spread evenly over the spinach, followed by the chopped tomatoes and fried eggs.

Whisk the vinaigrette ingredients together and serve with your salad. Store leftovers in an airtight container in the fridge for up to 3 days.

SERVES 4
PREP TIME: 10 MINUTES
COOKING TIME: 20 MINUTES

CALORIES: 432
CARBS: 10
PROTEIN: 17
FAT: 36

SOUTHWESTERN SCRAMBLE

A big ol' scramble is just the ticket, and this one is filled with veggies and healthy fats. We used pepper Jack cheese, but feel free to use any cheese that you have on hand!

2 tablespoons (30 g) butter

½ medium (75 g) yellow onion, sliced

2 garlic cloves, minced

1 medium (150 g) bell pepper (any color), seeded and sliced

1 teaspoon (5 g) sea salt

½ teaspoon (1 g) black pepper

1 teaspoon (5 g) red pepper flakes

6 large eggs

½ cup (56 g) shredded pepper Jack cheese

GARNISH:

Minced fresh cilantro

1 medium (150 g) avocado, peeled, pitted, and diced

2 tablespoons (30 g) full-fat sour cream

Salsa or hot sauce

INSTRUCTIONS:

Melt the butter in a cast-iron skillet over medium heat. Add the onion and garlic and sauté until soft, about 5 minutes.

Add the bell pepper, sea salt, black pepper, and red pepper flakes and continue to sauté until soft, about 5 minutes.

Crack the eggs into the pan and quickly scramble them, cooking until done to your desired preference. When done, sprinkle the shredded cheese over the entire skillet and cover the skillet so that the cheese melts. Serve, garnishing each serving with fresh cilantro, diced avocado, 1 tablespoon sour cream, and your favorite salsa or hot sauce.

SERVES 2
PREP TIME: 10 MINUTES
COOKING TIME: 15 MINUTES

CALORIES: 573
CARBS: 6
PROTEIN: 27
FAT: 48

BUTTERNUT AND LOX SCRAMBLE

A big everything bagel with cream cheese and lox is tasty, yes, but our version as a scramble will help you feel your best without compromising on flavor. Creamy roasted butternut squash is paired with salty, smoked salmon for a mouthwatering scramble to keep you feeling satisfied and energized.

BUTTERNUT SQUASH:

- 4 **cups (500 g) cubed butternut squash**
- 2 **tablespoons (30 g) butter, cut into small pieces**
- 1 **teaspoon (5 g) sea salt**
- ½ **teaspoon (1 g) black pepper**

EGGS:

- 1 **tablespoon (15 g) butter**
- 8 **large eggs**
- 1 **teaspoon (5 g) sea salt**
- ½ **teaspoon (1 g) black pepper**
- 1 **scallion, sliced**
- 4 **ounces (114 g) cream cheese, cut into small pieces**
- 4 **ounces (114 g) smoked salmon, torn into bite-size pieces**

GARNISH:

Minced fresh parsley

INSTRUCTIONS:

Preheat the oven to 350°F (180°C). Line a rimmed baking sheet with parchment paper.

Spread out the cubed butternut squash on the prepared baking sheet. Scatter the butter pieces over the squash and season with the sea salt and black pepper. Bake until the squash is soft and beginning to brown around the edges, about 25 minutes. Remove from the oven and set aside.

To make the eggs, melt the butter in a skillet over medium heat. When the butter is sizzling, crack each egg into the pan and quickly scramble (it will not look like perfect scrambled eggs, but it will taste delicious). Season the eggs with the sea salt, black pepper, and sliced scallion and continue to scramble.

When the eggs are done to your liking, turn off the heat and add the cream cheese and smoked salmon to the skillet. Cover and allow the cream cheese to melt a bit.

Top with fresh parsley and serve together with the butternut squash preparation.

SERVES 4	CALORIES: 451
PREP TIME: 15 MINUTES	CARBS: 23
COOKING TIME: 35 MINUTES	PROTEIN: 22
	FAT: 33

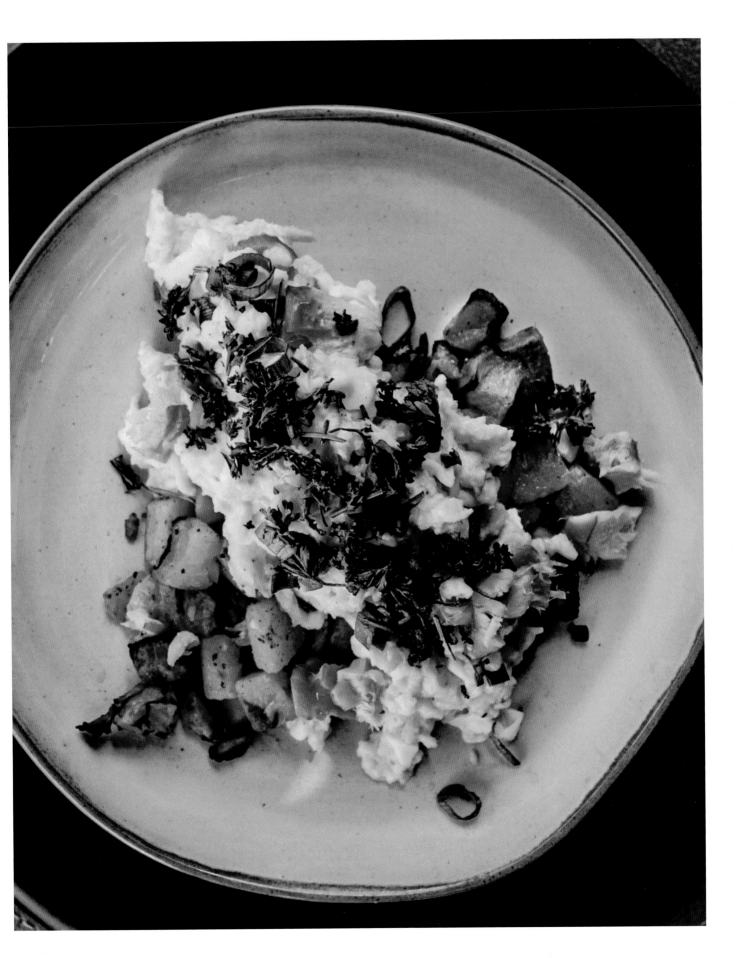

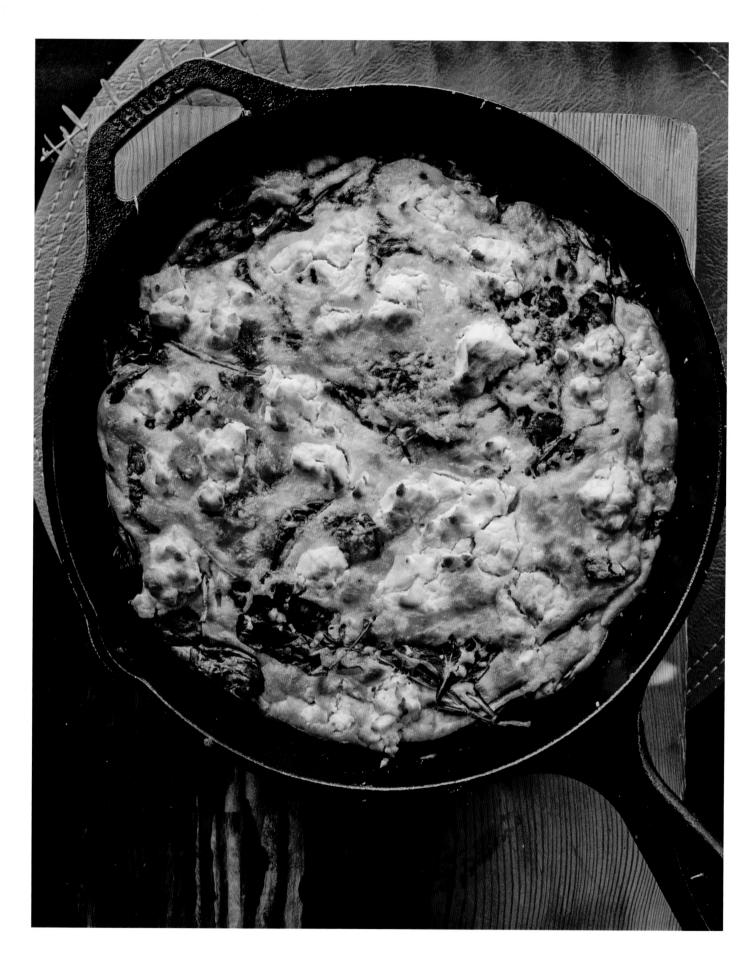

BUTTERNUT AND GOAT CHEESE FRITTATA

Roasted butternut squash makes this frittata extra creamy and offers a hint of natural sweetness. Paired with tangy sour cream, mouthwatering goat cheese, and fresh baby spinach, this is a dish you'll want to make over and over. We love ours served with a side of thick-cut bacon and some hot coffee!

BUTTERNUT SQUASH:

- **4 cups (500 g) cubed butternut squash**
- **2 tablespoons (30 g) butter, cut into small pieces**
- **1 teaspoon (5 g) sea salt**
- **½ teaspoon (1 g) black pepper**

EGGS:

- **8 large eggs**
- **¼ cup (60 g) full-fat sour cream**
- **1 teaspoon (5 g) sea salt**
- **½ teaspoon (1 g) black pepper**
- **Pinch ground nutmeg**
- **4 cups (120 g) baby spinach, chopped**
- **2 garlic cloves, minced**
- **Grated zest of ½ lemon**
- **4 ounces (114 g) goat cheese, cut into small pieces**

INSTRUCTIONS:

Preheat the oven to 350°F (180°C). Line a rimmed baking sheet with parchment paper.

Spread out the cubed butternut squash on the prepared baking sheet. Scatter the butter pieces over the squash and season with the sea salt and black pepper. Bake until the squash is soft and beginning to brown around the edges, about 25 minutes.

While the squash is baking, whisk the eggs in a large mixing bowl. Whisk in the sour cream, followed by the sea salt, black pepper, ground nutmeg, spinach, garlic, and lemon zest.

When the squash is done, remove it from the oven and transfer to an 8-inch cast-iron skillet.

Pour the egg mixture over the squash and scatter the goat cheese on top. Bake until the top is lightly browned, 30–35 minutes.

Remove from the oven and serve.

SERVES 4

PREP TIME: 15 MINUTES

COOKING TIME: 50 MINUTES

CALORIES: 383

CARBS: 24

PROTEIN: 21

FAT: 24

RADISH HASH WITH FRIED EGGS

Radishes are the star in this breakfast hash, and we love how they replace high-carb potatoes so easily! Boiling them for up to a minute prior to frying is an important step, so don't skip this part. A drizzle of olive oil added at the end of cooking ensures that each serving has enough fats.

RADISHES:

- ½ **pound (228 g) radishes**
- 2 **tablespoons (30 g) butter**
- 1 **teaspoon (5 g) sea salt**
- ½ **teaspoon (1 g) black pepper**
- ½ **teaspoon (0.7 g) garlic powder**
- 1 **teaspoon (5 g) dried rosemary**

EGGS:

- 1 **tablespoon (15 g) butter**
- 4 **large eggs**
- ½ **teaspoon (2.5 g) sea salt**

GARNISH:

- 2 **tablespoons (30 mL) extra-virgin olive oil**
- **Minced fresh parsley**

INSTRUCTIONS:

Fill a large saucepan with water and bring to a boil. Add the radishes and boil briefly, 30–60 seconds, and transfer to a bowl using a slotted spoon. When cool enough to handle, chop the radishes.

Melt the butter in a large cast-iron skillet over medium-high heat. When hot, add the radishes, sea salt, black pepper, garlic powder, and rosemary. Cook, turning only once or twice, until golden-brown, about 8 minutes.

Push the radish mixture to the sides of the skillet, melt 1 tablespoon butter in the center, and add the eggs, salting each individually. For over-easy eggs, cook uncovered for 4–6 minutes; for over-medium eggs, cover the pan and cook for 3 minutes, then uncover and continue cooking just until the whites are set, 2–3 minutes longer.

Serve the fried eggs over the radishes, garnishing each serving with 1 tablespoon olive oil and minced parsley.

SERVES **2**
PREP TIME: **5 MINUTES**
COOKING TIME: **15 MINUTES**

CALORIES: **452**
CARBS: **7**
PROTEIN: **12**
FAT: **41**

CHEESE AND GREEN CHILE CHICKEN AND EGG CASSEROLE

Whip this up when you have family in town for an extra-satisfying keto brunch, full of protein and healthy fat. Garnish with your favorite toppings, such as salsa, sour cream, and diced jalapeños!

- 2 tablespoons (30 g) butter
- 8 large eggs
- 1 (4-ounce/113 g) can diced green chiles
- 1 teaspoon (5 g) sea salt
- ½ teaspoon (1 g) black pepper
- ½ teaspoon (0.7 g) garlic powder
- 2 cups (500 g) cottage cheese, drained well
- 1 cup (140 g) chopped cooked chicken breast
- 2 cups (228 g) shredded extra-sharp Cheddar cheese
- 1 medium (150 g) avocado, peeled, pitted, and halved
- ½ cup (90 g) canned sliced black olives
- 1 scallion, minced

INSTRUCTIONS:

Preheat the oven to 350°F (180°C). Butter an 8-inch square baking dish.

Whisk the eggs in a mixing bowl and pour into the prepared baking dish. Add the green chiles (no need to drain), followed by the sea salt, black pepper, and garlic powder. Add the cottage cheese and gently mix into the eggs.

Add the chicken on top, followed by the shredded cheese, diced avocado, and sliced black olives.

Bake until the cheese is melted and the eggs are cooked through, 20–25 minutes.

Garnish with the scallion and allow to cool for a few minutes before serving.

SERVES 4
PREP TIME: 10 MINUTES
COOKING TIME: 30 MINUTES

CALORIES: 666
CARBS: 9
PROTEIN: 48
FAT: 47

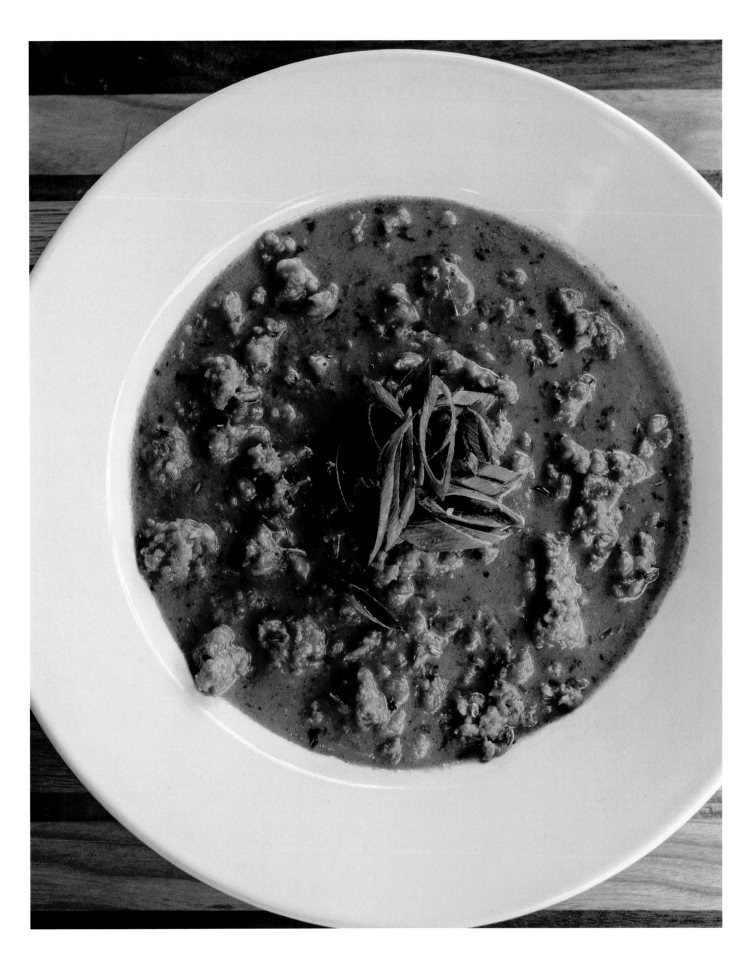

COWBOY SAUSAGE GRAVY

Truthfully, real cowboys are not making this gravy, but that's only because they're too busy roping up cattle to have ordered coconut milk and almond butter online. Help a cowboy out and let them know about this recipe for gravy as soon as you can and the world will be a much better place. This will store nicely for a couple of weeks in the fridge, making for an exciting and ready-made accompaniment to a variety of meals, especially eggs.

1 tablespoon (15 g) ghee or butter

1 pound (454 g) ground pork

½ (13.5-ounce/398 mL) can full-fat coconut milk

1 teaspoon (5 g) smoked paprika

1 teaspoon (5 g) dried oregano

1 teaspoon (5 g) fennel seeds

Sea salt and black pepper to taste

2 tablespoons (32 g) creamy almond butter

Sliced scallion greens, for garnish

INSTRUCTIONS:

Melt the ghee in a large skillet over medium heat. Add the pork and cook, breaking it up with a wooden spoon. Once the pork is cooked through, add the canned coconut milk (no need to drain the pork grease because this is cowboy-style, remember), smoked paprika, oregano, fennel seeds, sea salt, and black pepper. Stir in the almond butter, garnish with scallion greens, and serve.

SERVES 2
PREP TIME: 10 MINUTES
COOKING TIME: 20 MINUTES

CALORIES: 559
CARBS: 5
PROTEIN: 24
FAT: 48

CREAMY SCRAMBLED EGGS

People think you need to whisk eggs in a bowl before scrambling, but that takes time and just dirties another bowl, so simply crack them into the pan and mix up with a spatula. A big spoonful of mayo makes these better than plain ol' eggs.

1 **teaspoon (5 g) ghee or butter**

3 **large eggs**

Sea salt and black pepper to taste

2 **tablespoons (30 g) Primal Kitchen avocado mayonnaise**

INSTRUCTIONS:

Melt the ghee in a large skillet set over medium heat. Crack the eggs into the skillet and scramble. Season with sea salt and black pepper and cook until done to your liking. Top with the mayo and serve.

SERVES 1–2

PREP TIME: 2 MINUTES

COOKING TIME: 7 MINUTES

CALORIES: 455

CARBS: 3

PROTEIN: 18

FAT: 43

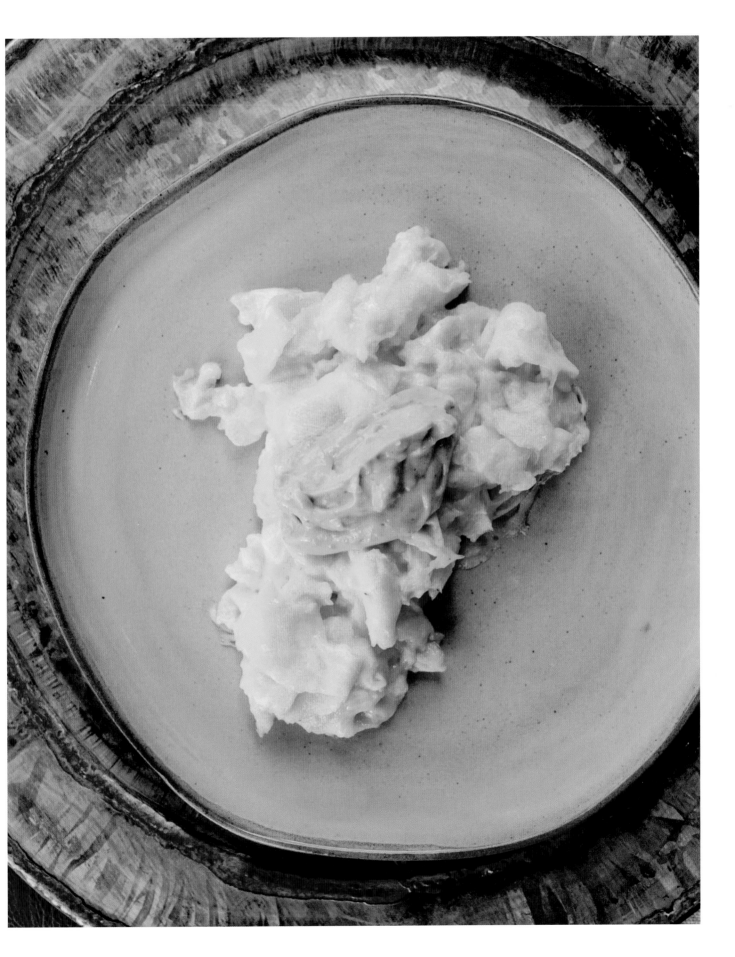

CLASSIC BREAKFAST PATTIES

Once you know that you can make really good-tasting breakfast sausage all by yourself, you'll take all of the other risks in life that you've been putting off. That might be a stretch, but it might not. Give it a try.

1 **pound (454 g) ground pork**

1 **teaspoon (1.25 g) garlic powder**

1 **tablespoon (6 g) fennel seeds**

Sea salt and black pepper to taste

INSTRUCTIONS:

In a large bowl, use your hands to gently mix the ground pork, garlic powder, fennel seeds, sea salt, and black pepper. Form the mixture into 8 patties.

Heat a large skillet over medium-high heat. Cook the patties until no longer pink, about 5 minutes per side.

SERVES 4–8

PREP TIME: **10 MINUTES**

COOKING TIME: **10 MINUTES**

CALORIES: **152**

CARBS: **1**

PROTEIN: **10**

FAT: **12**

CORNED BEEF BREAKFAST SKILLET

We think that most people make a big corned beef so that they can add it to scrambles the next day, but we're biased (but willing to talk about it). In a pinch, and that's how it is for us most days, you can use deli pastrami and ditch the caraway seeds if it's too annoying to find them at the grocery store (hint: they're located in the spice aisle). Serve on its own or with fried eggs.

1 tablespoon (15 g) ghee or butter

6 ounces (170 g) corned beef or deli pastrami, chopped

1 medium (160 g) onion, chopped

1 large (150 g) bell pepper (any color), chopped

½ teaspoon (1 g) caraway seeds

Sea salt, black pepper, and garlic powder to taste

INSTRUCTIONS:

Melt the ghee in a large cast-iron skillet set to medium-high heat. Add the corned beef, onion, and bell pepper and season with the caraway seeds, sea salt, black pepper, and garlic powder. Cook, tossing every now and then, until everything has browned, about 10 minutes.

SERVES 2
PREP TIME: 10 MINUTES
COOKING TIME: 20 MINUTES

CALORIES: 239
CARBS: 12
PROTEIN: 21
FAT: 11

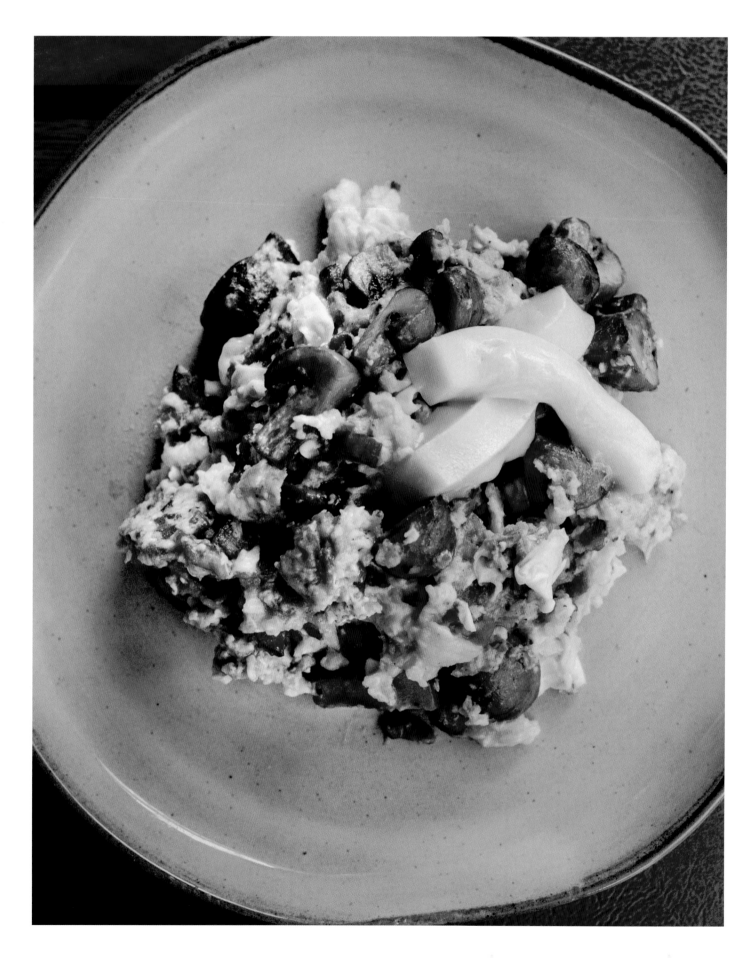

BACON AND MUSHROOM SCRAMBLE

If you need to impress someone, just buy Brie cheese. Done. But to really impress, make this scramble. It's the perfect combination of texture and flavor and increases your cool factor by a good 10 percent each time you serve it.

6 **bacon strips**

1 **cup (75 g) cremini mushrooms, quartered or halved**

Sea salt and black pepper to taste

4 **large eggs**

2 **ounces (56 g) Brie cheese, broken up into pieces**

INSTRUCTIONS:

Cook the bacon in a cast-iron skillet over medium heat until crispy, 5–7 minutes. Transfer the bacon to a plate, leaving the grease in the skillet.

Add the mushrooms to the skillet, season with sea salt and black pepper, and cook, tossing occasionally, until soft, about 3 minutes.

Crack the eggs into the skillet, season with sea salt and black pepper, and begin scrambling. It's okay for the whites and yolks to cook somewhat separately; you'll appreciate the distinct flavors in your scramble when it's on your plate—and in your mouth!

Transfer the eggs to a plate, top with the Brie, and serve.

SERVES 2

PREP TIME: 5 MINUTES

COOKING TIME: 20 MINUTES

CALORIES: 756

CARBS: 6

PROTEIN: 54

FAT: 58

CURRIED CAULIFLOWER EGG BAKE

Sometimes it's necessary to make an impressive breakfast, and this is just one way to do that. A bit unexpected for morning, but that's the whole point. You will really impress by adding some fresh herbs to this after it's out of the oven. You're welcome.

1 **pound (454 g) cauliflower florets**

1 **tablespoon (15 g) ghee or butter**

Sea salt and black pepper to taste

1 **tablespoon (7 g) curry powder**

4 **large eggs**

Minced fresh parsley, cilantro, or chives, for garnish

INSTRUCTIONS:

Preheat the oven to 400°F (200°C).

In an ovenproof skillet, toss the cauliflower florets with the ghee, sea salt, black pepper, and curry powder. Bake until soft, about 20 minutes, tossing after 10 minutes.

Crack the eggs over the cauliflower and bake until the egg whites are cooked through, about 7 minutes more. Fancy this up with some fresh herbs on top.

SERVES 2
PREP TIME: 5 MINUTES
COOKING TIME: 25 MINUTES

CALORIES: 278
CARBS: 16
PROTEIN: 16
FAT: 17

DRY OATMEAL

This oatmeal preparation is the fastest breakfast or post-workout snack you can imagine. It has an interesting mix of flavors and distinct textures. It will also "stick to your bones" like Grandma's oatmeal, but without the insulin spike. If you can't find coconut butter at your grocery store, puree some coconut flakes in a blender.

- 1 tablespoon (15 g) coconut butter
- 2 tablespoons (30 g) almond butter or peanut butter
- 2 tablespoons (30 g) cacao nibs
- 2 tablespoons (12 g) unsweetened shredded coconut
- ⅓ cup (80 mL) unsweetened full-fat coconut milk or almond milk

  Pomegranate seeds, for topping (optional)

INSTRUCTIONS:

In a bowl, mash together the coconut butter, almond butter, cacao nibs, and shredded coconut to a paste consistency. Add the milk and stir to make a porridge. Top with pomegranate seeds if you like and enjoy cold.

SERVES 1

PREP TIME: 10 MINUTES

CALORIES: 444

CARBS: 18

PROTEIN: 11

FAT: 39

COLD KETO BREAKFAST PLATE FOR A HOT SUMMER DAY

Some days it's too hot to cook even the quickest meal, so may we introduce to you the cold keto plate to save the day. It's better for you than cereal, and ideal to prepare when you're out of leftovers to serve for breakfast.

½ medium (75 g) avocado, peeled and pitted

Lime juice to taste

Sea salt and black pepper to taste

2 large soft- or hard-boiled eggs, peeled and cut into wedges

5 cherry tomatoes (85 g), halved

¼ cup (2 g) chopped fresh cilantro or scallion (optional)

INSTRUCTIONS:

Mash up the avocado with lime juice, sea salt, and black pepper. A fork or potato masher both work well for this. Serve with eggs and halved cherry tomatoes. Amp this up with some fresh cilantro or scallion.

SERVES 1
PREP TIME: 10 MINUTES

CALORIES: 277
CARBS: 11
PROTEIN: 14
FAT: 21

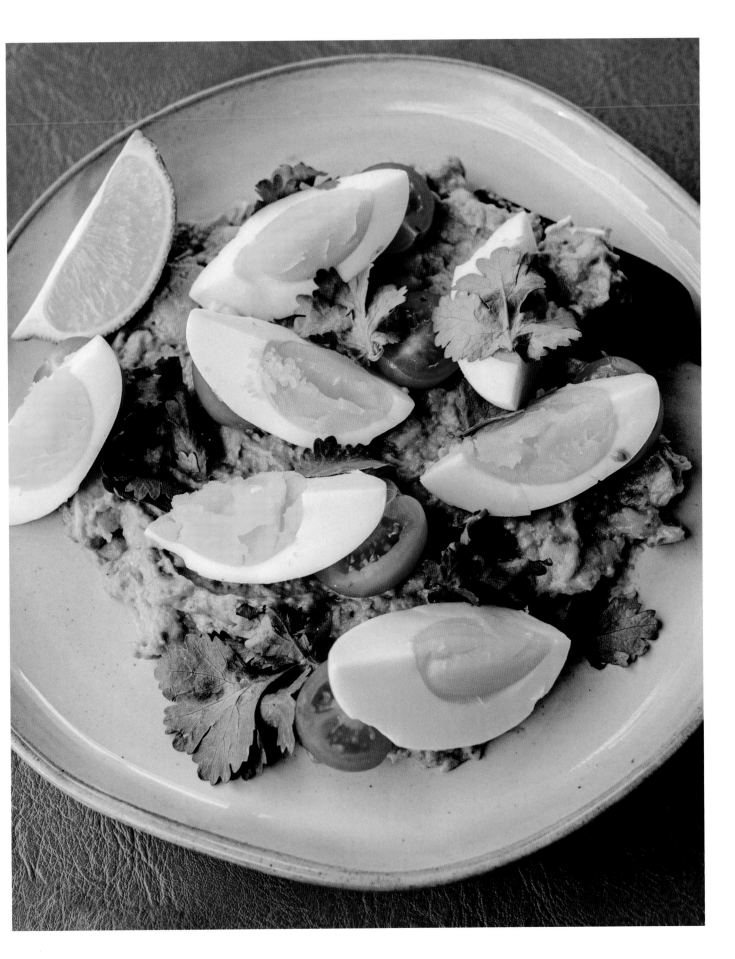

NORI BREAKFAST BURRITO

Nori makes for a great tortilla substitute, especially when used with eggs since the moisture helps soften and seal the nori wrap together. We like to hide nutrient-dense braunschweiger sausage in our "noritos."

4 **ounces (113 g) braunschweiger sausage**

5 **large eggs**

Ghee or coconut oil (optional)

8 **nori sheets**

2 **tablespoons (30 mL) Tapatío or Cholula hot sauce**

INSTRUCTIONS:

Cook the sausage in a skillet until browned. Depending on what kind of sausage you use, it might have enough fat content to cook itself and the eggs; if not, add some ghee or coconut oil.

Crack the eggs into the skillet and scramble. Remove from the heat.

On your countertop, lay out 4 nori sheets in a big square, overlapping in the middle. Then lay out the other 4 in the same way.

Pour half of the eggs and sausage down the middle of each nori square and wrap like a burrito.

Serve with a few dashes of hot sauce per your preference.

SERVES 2
PREP TIME: 10 MINUTES
COOKING TIME: 5 MINUTES

CALORIES: 403
CARBS: 8
PROTEIN: 27
FAT: 30

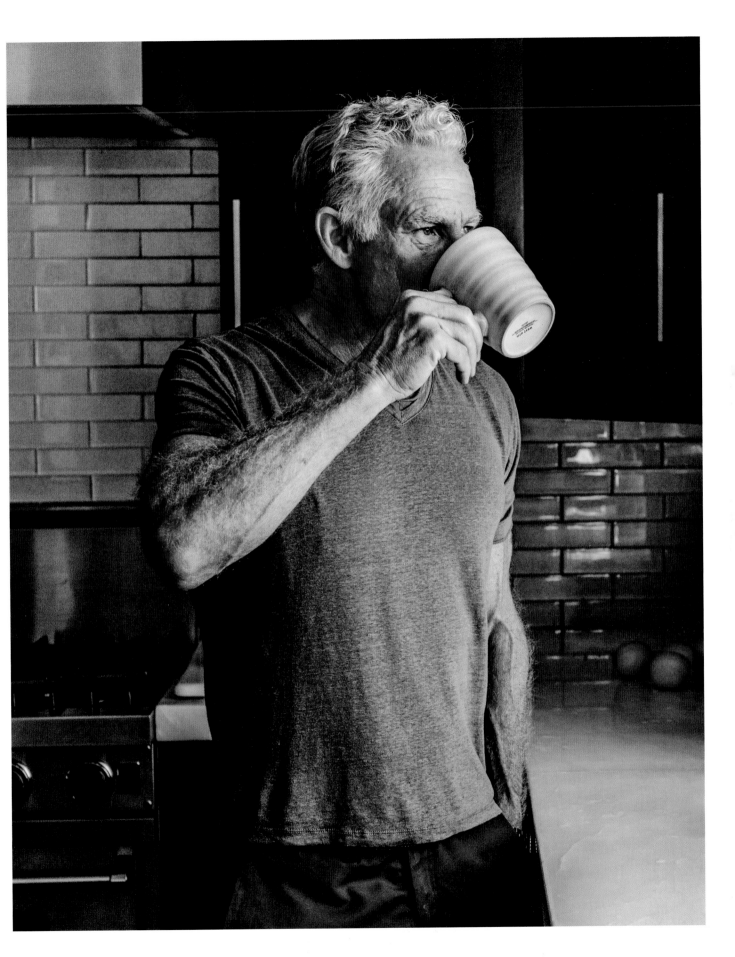

SAVORY APPE-TIZERS

CHAPTER 5

Meatballs and more that are great to have around when you want something substantial but don't have time to prepare a proper meal. These preparations will be the talk of the party potluck too!

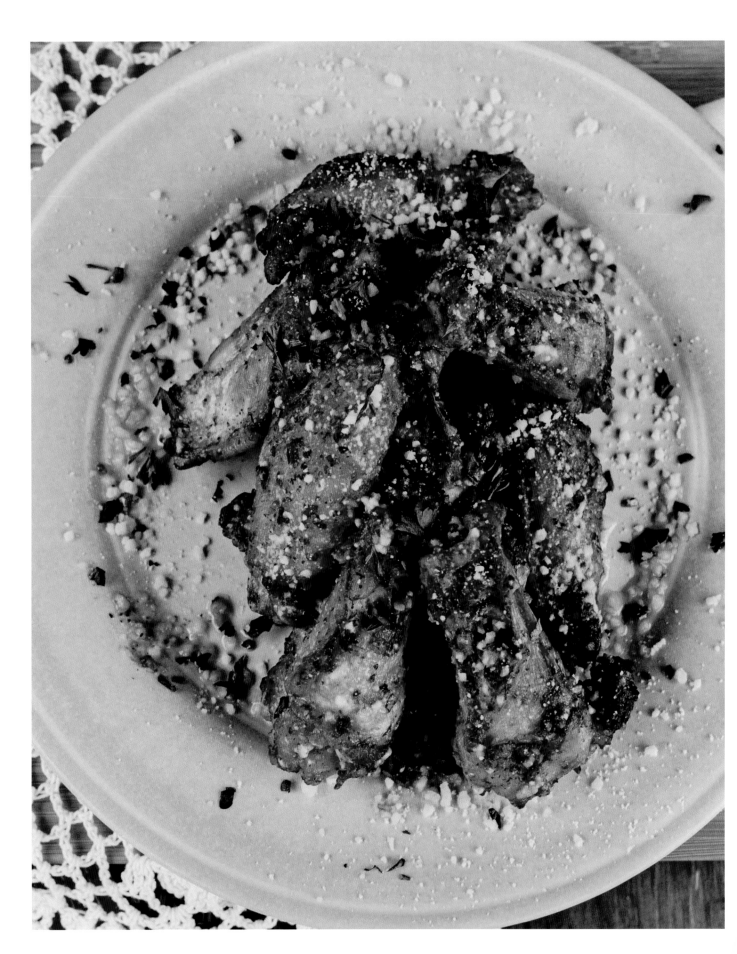

GARLIC AND PARMESAN CHICKEN WINGS

These chicken wings are extra flavorful thanks to the garlic and Parmesan. Dip them in high-quality ranch dressing to ensure maximum nutrition.

- **1 pound (454 g) chicken wings**
- **4 tablespoons (60 g) butter, divided**
- **1 teaspoon (5 g) sea salt**
- **½ teaspoon (1 g) black pepper**
- **6 garlic cloves, minced**
- **½ cup (120 mL) ranch dressing**
- **½ cup (50 g) grated Parmesan cheese**
- **¼ cup (16 g) chopped fresh parsley, for garnish**

INSTRUCTIONS:

Preheat the oven to 400°F (200°C).

Pat dry the chicken wings to prepare them for cooking. Heat a cast-iron skillet over medium-high heat. When hot, place the chicken wings in the skillet and sear on both sides, about 2 minutes per side.

Add 2 tablespoons of the butter to the skillet and season the wings with sea salt and black pepper. Place the skillet in the oven to finish cooking the chicken wings, about 25 minutes.

Remove the skillet from the oven and return it to the stovetop over medium-high heat. Add the remaining 2 tablespoons butter and the garlic and sauté until the wings are coated and the garlic has turned golden.

Toss the wings with ranch dressing, sprinkle the Parmesan cheese on top of the wings, and remove the skillet from the heat. Serve hot, topped with some chopped parsley. Store leftovers in an airtight container in the fridge for up to 3 days.

SERVES 4
PREP TIME: 5 MINUTES
COOKING TIME: 30 MINUTES

CALORIES: 537
CARBS: 5
PROTEIN: 28
FAT: 45

CHEDDAR AND SWISS PORK MEATBALLS

Need something incredibly tasty to make right this moment? You've come to the right place! These meatballs are ultra-savory, with creamy Cheddar and Swiss cheese and fatty ground pork. You will be so glad you decided to make them!

- **1 pound (454 g) ground pork**
- **¼ cup (28 g) shredded Cheddar cheese**
- **¼ cup (28 g) shredded Swiss cheese**
- **1 large egg, whisked**
- **½ cup (60 g) almond flour**
- **½ cup (32 g) minced fresh parsley**
- **2 scallions, minced**
- **1 teaspoon (5 g) sea salt**
- **½ teaspoon (1 g) black pepper**
- **1 teaspoon (1.25 g) garlic powder**

INSTRUCTIONS:

Preheat the oven to 350°F (180°C). Line a rimmed baking sheet with parchment paper.

Combine all the ingredients in a large bowl and mix well with your hands or a large spoon. Form the mixture into 20 meatballs (about 1½ inches in diameter) and place on the prepared baking sheet.

Bake for 10 minutes, flip the meatballs with a pair of tongs, and continue baking until cooked through, another 5–8 minutes.

Let cool for a few minutes, then transfer to a serving plate. Serve with toothpicks inserted into each for easy grabbing. Store leftovers in the fridge for up to 3 days.

SERVES 10
PREP TIME: 10 MINUTES
COOKING TIME: 15 MINUTES

CALORIES: 176
CARBS: 2
PROTEIN: 11
FAT: 14

BACON AND CABBAGE STIR-FRY

Serve this easy stir-fry with some fried eggs, a seared steak, or a flaky piece of white fish. You are going to love its simple keto flavors!

- 8 **bacon strips**
- 2 **tablespoons (30 g) butter**
- 4 **garlic cloves, minced**
- 1 **pound (454 g) shredded green cabbage**
- 1 **teaspoon (5 g) sea salt**
- ½ **teaspoon (1 g) black pepper**

INSTRUCTIONS:

Cook the bacon in a skillet over medium heat until crispy, 5–7 minutes. Transfer the bacon to a plate, leaving the grease in the skillet.

Add the butter to the skillet and reduce the heat to medium-low. Add the garlic and cabbage and sauté until the cabbage is soft and the garlic is golden, about 5 minutes. Season with the sea salt and black pepper and continue to sauté until soft, about 3 more minutes.

Serve the cabbage stir-fry with the bacon. Store leftovers in an airtight container in the fridge for up to 3 days.

SERVES 4
PREP TIME: 5 MINUTES
COOKING TIME: 20 MINUTES

CALORIES: 161
CARBS: 7
PROTEIN: 7
FAT: 13

TERIYAKI MEATBALLS

These meatballs are bursting with fresh flavor from scallion, ginger, and savory coconut aminos. Serve with a side of riced cauliflower, roasted zucchini, steamed green beans, or sautéed peppers for a truly satisfying keto meal!

- 8 **ounces (228 g) ground pork**
- 1 **large egg, whisked**
- 2 **garlic cloves, minced**
- 1 **scallion, minced**
- 2 **teaspoons (10 g) minced fresh ginger**
- 1 **tablespoon (15 g) almond flour**
- 1 **teaspoon (5 g) sea salt**
- ½ **teaspoon (1 g) black pepper**
- 1 **teaspoon (5 g) red pepper flakes**
- 2 **tablespoons (8 g) chopped fresh cilantro**

GARNISH:

- 2 **tablespoons (30 mL) coconut aminos**
- 1 **tablespoon (15 mL) toasted sesame oil**
- 1 **tablespoon (15 g) sesame seeds**
- **Sliced scallion**

INSTRUCTIONS:

Preheat the oven to 400°F (200°C). Line a rimmed baking sheet with parchment paper.

Gently combine all the meatball ingredients in a mixing bowl until well combined. Form the mixture into 2-inch meatballs with your hands and arrange on the prepared baking sheet.

Bake until browned, about 15 minutes.

Drizzle plate with coconut aminos and sesame oil, and serve with a sprinkle of sesame seeds and sliced scallion.

SERVES 8
PREP TIME: 5 MINUTES
COOKING TIME: 15 MINUTES

CALORIES: 109
CARBS: 1
PROTEIN: 6
FAT: 9

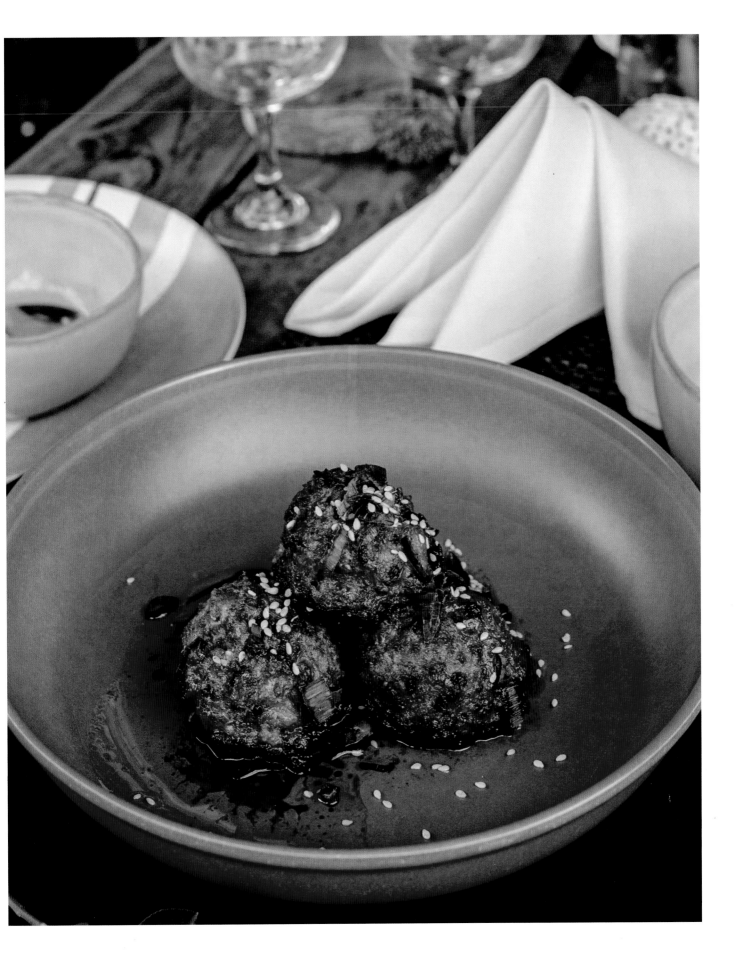

SWEDISH MEATBALLS

This warm and comforting dish is perfect to make and enjoy with loved ones or to have as leftovers throughout the week. If you don't tolerate dairy well, opt for coconut cream—you will love it just as much! Serve the meatballs on their own or over riced cauliflower or zucchini noodles.

MEATBALLS:

- 2 tablespoons (30 g) butter, divided
- ½ medium (150 g) yellow onion, minced
- 3 garlic cloves, minced
- 1 pound (454 g) ground beef
- 1 large egg, whisked
- 1 tablespoon (15 g) almond flour
- 1 teaspoon (5 g) sea salt
- ½ teaspoon (1 g) black pepper
- 1 teaspoon (5 g) red pepper flakes
- 1 teaspoon (5 g) Italian seasoning
- 1 teaspoon (5 g) pumpkin pie spice

SAUCE:

- 4 tablespoons (60 g) butter
- 1 tablespoon (15 g) almond flour
- 2 cups (480 mL) beef stock or bone broth
- 2 tablespoons (30 mL) coconut aminos
- 1 tablespoon (15 g) Dijon mustard
- Grated zest of ½ lemon
- 1 tablespoon (15 mL) fresh lemon juice
- 1 cup (240 mL) heavy cream or canned coconut cream

SERVES 8
PREP TIME: 15 MINUTES
COOKING TIME: 30 MINUTES

CALORIES: 346
CARBS: 5
PROTEIN: 13
FAT: 30

INSTRUCTIONS:

To make the meatballs, melt 1 tablespoon of the butter in a large skillet over medium-low heat. Add the minced onion and minced garlic and sauté until soft, about 5 minutes. Transfer the onion and garlic to a large bowl. Add the ground beef, egg, almond flour, sea salt, black pepper, red pepper flakes, Italian seasoning, and pumpkin pie spice and mix well. Form the mixture into 8 meatballs.

Melt the remaining 1 tablespoon butter in the same skillet over medium heat. Add the meatballs and sear until browned on all sides, about 3 minutes per side. Transfer the meatballs to a plate.

To make the sauce, melt the butter in the same skillet over medium heat. Add the almond flour and allow it to brown, stirring occasionally. Pour in the beef stock and whisk to combine. Add the coconut aminos, mustard, and lemon zest and juice and whisk well. Bring to a simmer and allow to thicken, about 15 minutes.

Stir in the cream and continue to simmer until very thick. Return the meatballs to the skillet, stir to coat in the sauce, and heat through. Serve hot.

ALMOND BUTTER CHICKEN

Almond butter is amazing on chicken. The end. Really, the next time you need a little something to tide you over, give this combo a try. It's sweet, salty, and creamy and really hits the spot.

2 **tablespoons (30 g) almond butter**

Sea salt and black pepper to taste

½ **cup (50 g) fresh blueberries**

6 **ounces (170 g) deli chicken or turkey slices**

INSTRUCTIONS:

Mix the almond butter in a bowl with a sprinkle of sea salt and black pepper. Fold in the blueberries.

Place a chicken slice on a cutting board and spread a small spoonful of the almond butter and blueberry mix onto the center. Flatten a little and roll it up. Repeat to make the remaining rolls.

SERVES **2**
PREP TIME: **10 MINUTES**
COOKING TIME: **10 MINUTES**

CALORIES: **201**
CARBS: **9**
PROTEIN: **20**
FAT: **11**

WALNUT HERB CHEESE LOG

This is the type of recipe that looks like it was more involved than it really was to prepare, so serve it for a party when you're looking to make a good impression. Just put it on a fancy platter and serve with in-season veggies, such as sliced cucumber, red bell peppers, or radish.

1 **cup (125 g) finely chopped walnuts**

2 **tablespoons (8 g) minced fresh parsley**

5 **dill sprigs, minced**

1 **scallion, minced**

Sea salt and black pepper to taste

1 **(1-pound/454 g) goat cheese log**

INSTRUCTIONS:

Toss the walnuts, parsley, dill, scallion, sea salt, and black pepper in a large bowl. Pour the mixture onto a flat surface (parchment paper works great) and roll the goat cheese log in it until the cheese is completely covered by walnuts and herbs.

SERVES 16

PREP TIME: 10 MINUTES

COOKING TIME: 5 MINUTES

CALORIES: 124

CARBS: 1

PROTEIN: 6

FAT: 11

SUN-DRIED TOMATO AND WALNUT DIP

If you like a textured dip bursting with flavor, this is the recipe you've been waiting for! We used dried basil, but by all means, use fresh if you have it. It's a pretty thick dip, so it actually works well to scoop it up with veggies or to serve it on top of grilled meats and fried eggs. Just top it with a big spoonful (2–3 tablespoons).

- 1 (8-ounce/241 g) jar sun-dried tomatoes packed in olive oil
- 1 cup (125 g) chopped walnuts
- 2 garlic cloves, peeled
- 1 tablespoon (2 g) dried basil or 1½ tablespoons (3 g) fresh basil leaves
- 1 tablespoon (15 mL) fresh lemon juice

  Sea salt and black pepper to taste

INSTRUCTIONS:

In a food processor, combine the sun-dried tomatoes (including the oil), walnuts, garlic cloves, basil, lemon juice, and a big sprinkle of sea salt and black pepper. Pulse until everything is minced, scraping down the sides of the processor bowl as needed.

SERVES 8
PREP TIME: 10 MINUTES
COOKING TIME: 10 MINUTES

CALORIES: 123
CARBS: 8
PROTEIN: 3
FAT: 10

BROCCOLI, BACON, AND AVOCADO MASH

When you're craving something creamy and fatty and don't care about anything else, you'll know you have gone keto. This recipe is delicious on its own but is also wonderful on a salad or with grilled meat. Add some red pepper flakes if you prefer a bit of heat.

4   bacon strips

1   medium (160 g) onion, chopped

     Sea salt, black pepper, and garlic powder to taste

1   pound (454 g) broccoli florets, chopped

2   medium (300 g) avocados, peeled and pitted

     Red pepper flakes (optional)

INSTRUCTIONS:

Cook the bacon in a skillet over medium heat until crispy, 5–7 minutes. Transfer the bacon to a plate, leaving the grease in the skillet.

Add the onion to the skillet and season with sea salt, black pepper, and garlic powder. Add the chopped broccoli, toss everything together, and cook until it has all softened and begins to caramelize, about 5 minutes.

Transfer the contents of the skillet to a food processor, add the avocados, and pulse until creamy. Crumble the bacon on top, season with red pepper flakes if desired, and serve.

SERVES 4

PREP TIME: 10 MINUTES

COOKING TIME: 15 MINUTES

CALORIES: 208

CARBS: 9

PROTEIN: 8

FAT: 16

CHICKEN AND TURKEY ENTREES

CHAPTER 6

Gone are the days when we eat chicken and broccoli and are terribly hungry and bored afterward, so if you're experiencing any traumatic flashbacks to old diets, take heart. In this section we emphasize the highest-quality proteins, and they are always paired with healthy fats to nourish and satisfy your wellness needs. Get ready to dig in and be rewarded with flavor and ease of preparation!

PESTO-STUFFED CHICKEN BREASTS

Creamy savory pesto is amazing baked inside juicy chicken breasts. Consider doubling or tripling the recipe to make for a party crowd—it's sure to please!

PESTO:

- ⅓ cup (80 mL) extra-virgin olive oil
- 1½ cups (50 g) basil leaves
- 2 tablespoons (16 g) pine nuts
- 2 garlic cloves, roughly chopped
- Grated zest and juice of ½ lemon
- 1 teaspoon (5 g) sea salt
- ½ teaspoon (1 g) black pepper

STUFFED CHICKEN BREASTS:

- 3 cups (300 g) cauliflower florets
- 1 tablespoon (3.75 g) garlic powder
- 1 teaspoon (5 g) sea salt
- ½ teaspoon (1 g) black pepper
- Pinch cayenne pepper
- 2 (4-ounce/228 g) boneless, skinless chicken breasts
- 3 tablespoons (45 g) ghee or butter

INSTRUCTIONS:

Preheat the oven to 350°F (180°C). Line a rimmed baking sheet with parchment paper.

To make the pesto, combine all the pesto ingredients in a blender or food processor and blend until creamy. Reserve 2 tablespoons to stuff the chicken breasts; store the remaining pesto in the fridge for up to 3 days.

To make the stuffed chicken breasts, pour an inch or two of water into a small saucepan with a steamer basket insert. Cover and bring to a boil over medium-high heat. Add the cauliflower florets to the steamer basket, cover, and steam until tender, about 10 minutes. Drain and transfer to a bowl. Add the reserved pesto and mash it together with the cauliflower. Set aside.

In a small bowl, mix together the garlic powder, sea salt, black pepper, and cayenne. Rub the mixture all over each chicken breast. Cut a slit in the thick side of each chicken breast so there's an opening to stuff the pesto mixture into it.

Melt the ghee in a large skillet set over medium heat. Add the chicken breasts and cook until slightly browned, about 5 minutes per side. Transfer the chicken to a plate.

When the chicken is cool enough to handle, spoon the cauliflower and pesto mixture into the slit of each chicken breast, then place on the prepared baking sheet. Bake until the chicken is fully cooked and has reached 165°F (75°C), about 20 minutes.

Serve hot. Store leftovers in an airtight container in the fridge for up to 3 days.

SERVES 2
PREP TIME: 5 MINUTES
COOKING TIME: 40 MINUTES

CALORIES: 721
CARBS: 8
PROTEIN: 50
FAT: 55

SHEET PAN CHICKEN THIGHS WITH ARTICHOKE HEARTS

Sheet pan meals make cooking easy-peasy, so invest in a large rimmed baking sheet to whip up recipes bursting with flavor, such as this chicken dish featuring artichoke hearts, lemon, and herbs.

- 8 (4-ounce/228 g) bone-in, skin-on chicken thighs
- 4 garlic cloves, minced
- 4 medium (248 g) zucchini, trimmed and sliced
- 2 (14-ounce/397 g) cans quartered artichoke hearts packed in water, drained
- 1 lemon, sliced and seeded
- ½ cup (114 g) butter, cut into small pieces
- ½ cup (120 mL) extra-virgin olive oil
- 4 teaspoons (20 g) sea salt
- 2 teaspoons (4 g) black pepper
- 2 tablespoons (30 g) dried tarragon
- 1 tablespoon (15 g) dried rosemary

GARNISH:

- ½ cup (32 g) minced fresh parsley
- 2 tablespoons (15 g) capers

INSTRUCTIONS:

Preheat the oven to 400°F (200°C). Line a rimmed baking sheet with parchment paper.

Arrange the chicken thighs, garlic, zucchini, artichoke hearts, and lemon slices on the prepared baking sheet.

Scatter the butter pieces on top of everything and then drizzle with the olive oil. Season everything with the sea salt, black pepper, dried tarragon, and dried rosemary.

Bake until the chicken reaches 165°F (75°C), 35–45 minutes. Garnish with fresh parsley and capers and serve.

SERVES 8
PREP TIME: 10 MINUTES
COOKING TIME: 40 MINUTES

CALORIES: 314
CARBS: 6
PROTEIN: 21
FAT: 23

CHICKEN POTPIE WITH CAULIFLOWER CRUST

This recipe features all the warm and comforting flavors of traditional chicken potpie without the excess carbs and grains. Make a big batch of this and share with loved ones—we know you're going to love it!

- 4 cups (400 g) riced cauliflower
- 1 cup (135 g) extra-sharp Cheddar cheese, divided
- 1 large egg, whisked
- 1 teaspoon (5 g) sea salt, divided
- ½ teaspoon (1 g) black pepper, divided
- 4 bacon strips

- 1 (150 g) medium yellow onion, diced
- 4 garlic cloves, minced
- 2 medium (100 g) carrots, peeled and diced
- 4 medium (200 g) celery stalks, diced
- 1 teaspoon (5 g) dried rosemary
- 1 teaspoon (5 g) dried thyme

- 1 pound (454 g) boneless, skinless chicken breasts, cut into bite-size pieces
- ½ cup (80 g) frozen peas
- 1 cup (70 g) sliced cremini mushrooms
- 1 cup (240 mL) chicken broth
- ½ cup (120 mL) heavy cream
- Minced fresh parsley, for garnish

SERVES 4

PREP TIME: 15 MINUTES

COOKING TIME: 50 MINUTES

CALORIES: 421

CARBS: 17

PROTEIN: 16

FAT: 32

INSTRUCTIONS:

Preheat the oven to 120°F (50°C). Line a rimmed baking sheet with parchment paper.

Put the riced cauliflower in a microwave-safe bowl and microwave for 5 minutes on high. Set aside to cool completely, about 10 minutes.

Place a paper towel over the riced cauliflower and squeeze out as much water as possible to ensure that it crisps during the cooking process. Spread out the riced cauliflower on the prepared baking sheet. Bake for 5 minutes. Stir and continue baking for another 5 minutes. Remove the baking sheet from the oven. Increase the oven temperature to 400°F (200°C).

Transfer the riced cauliflower to a bowl. Add ½ cup of the Cheddar cheese, followed by the egg, ½ teaspoon of the sea salt, and ¼ teaspoon of the black pepper and mix until completely combined. Press the mixture into the bottom and partway up the edges of an 8-inch round nonstick baking pan to form a crust. Bake until browned, about 25 minutes.

Meanwhile, cook the bacon in a skillet over medium heat until crispy, 5–7 minutes. Transfer the bacon to a plate, leaving the grease in the skillet.

Add the onion, garlic, carrots, and celery to the grease remaining in the skillet and cook over medium-high heat until softened, about 5 minutes. After adding the onion and other veggies and before adding the chicken, season with rosemary and thyme. Add the chicken and cook until cooked through, about 5 minutes. Add the peas and mushrooms and cook until the mushrooms have softened and the peas are heated through, about 5 minutes.

Pour the chicken broth and cream into the skillet. Season with the remaining ½ teaspoon sea salt and remaining ¼ teaspoon black pepper and stir well. Reduce the heat and simmer until the sauce has reduced by one-fourth, about 5 minutes.

Pour the chicken mixture into the prebaked cauliflower crust. Crumble the bacon into medium bits and sprinkle it on top of the mixture, along with the remaining ½ cup Cheddar cheese.

Switch the oven to broil. Place the chicken potpie under the broiler until browned and bubbling, 5–10 minutes. Allow to cool for about 5 minutes, garnish with the parsley, and serve. Store leftovers in the fridge for up to 3 days.

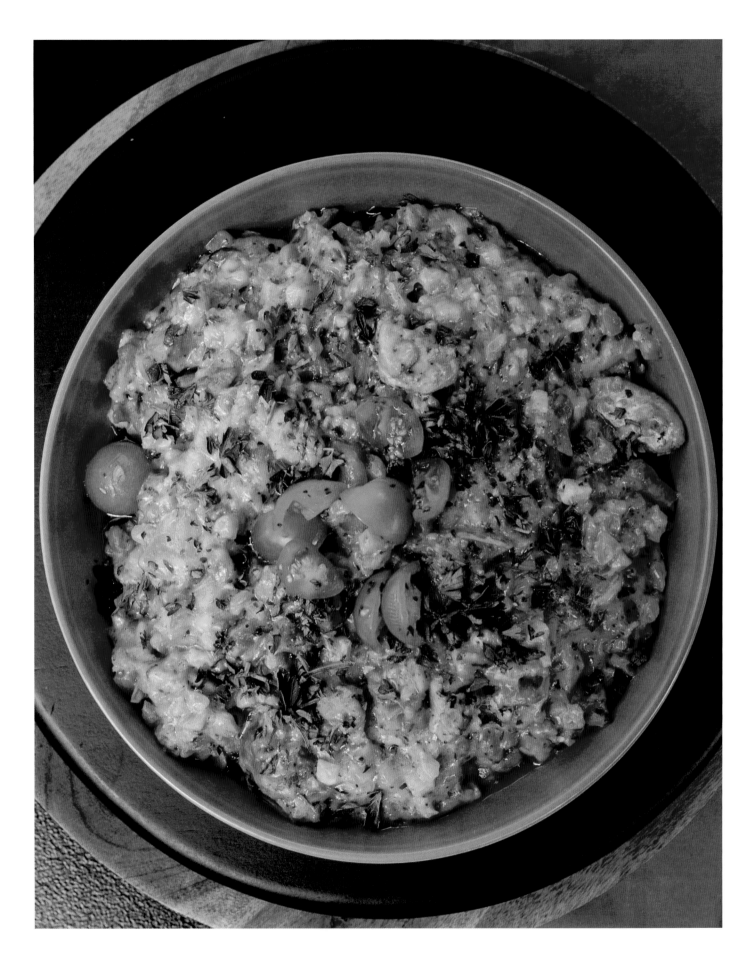

KETO CHICKEN SKILLET

This skillet meal combines protein and veggies in a creamy sauce that will have your mouth watering. Garnish with fresh parsley, scallion, or grated lemon zest to brighten it up even more!

- 2 **tablespoons (30 g) butter**
- 1 **medium (150 g) yellow onion, chopped**
- 2 **garlic cloves, minced**
- 1 **teaspoon (5 g) sea salt**
- ½ **teaspoon (1 g) black pepper**
- 1 **tablespoon (15 g) dried Italian seasoning**
- 1 **pound (454 g) boneless, skinless chicken thighs, cut into bite-size pieces**
- 4 **cups (400 g) riced cauliflower**
- 4 **tablespoons (60 g) cream cheese**
- 2 **cups (228 g) shredded Cheddar cheese**
- 1 **cup (150 g) cherry tomatoes, quartered**

INSTRUCTIONS:

Melt the butter in a Dutch oven or large soup pot over medium-low heat. Add the onion and garlic and sauté until soft, about 5 minutes. Season with sea salt, black pepper, and Italian seasoning and stir well to combine.

Add the chicken and cook until browned, stirring often, about 10 minutes. Stir in the riced cauliflower and sauté until warmed through, about 5 minutes. Turn off the heat and stir in the cream cheese and shredded cheese. Top with the cherry tomatoes and serve hot. Store leftovers in an airtight container in the fridge for up to 3 days.

SERVES 4
PREP TIME: 15 MINUTES
COOKING TIME: 20 MINUTES

CALORIES: 451
CARBS: 12
PROTEIN: 34
FAT: 28

EASY CHICKEN SOUP

Chicken soup warms the heart and nourishes the body any time of the year. We add diced avocado to ours to increase the healthy fats, and a sprinkle of good-quality cheese would be delicious, too!

- 4 **tablespoons (60 g) butter**
- 1 **medium (150 g) yellow onion, chopped**
- 3 **garlic cloves, minced**
- 1 **teaspoon (5 g) sea salt**
- ½ **teaspoon (1 g) black pepper**
- 1 **teaspoon (5 g) dried thyme**
- 2 **medium (100 g) carrots, peeled and diced**
- 4 **medium (200 g) celery stalks, diced**
- 4 **cups (400 g) cauliflower florets**
- 4 **cups (960 mL) chicken broth**
- 1 **pound (454 g) boneless, skinless chicken breasts, cut into bite-size pieces**
- 1 **medium (150 g) avocado, peeled, pitted, and diced**

  Minced fresh parsley, for garnish

INSTRUCTIONS:

Melt the butter in a Dutch oven or large soup pot over medium-low heat. Add the onion and garlic and sauté until soft, about 5 minutes. Season with the sea salt, black pepper, and thyme and stir well to combine.

Add the carrots, celery, cauliflower florets, and chicken broth and bring to a simmer. Stir in the chicken breast and continue to simmer for 15 minutes.

Remove the pan from the heat and stir in the avocado. Garnish with fresh parsley and serve. Store leftovers in an airtight container in the fridge for up to 3 days.

SERVES 4
PREP TIME: 15 MINUTES
COOKING TIME: 25 MINUTES

CALORIES: 397
CARBS: 9
PROTEIN: 40
FAT: 22

CHICKEN RANCH SOUP

This soup is ultra-creamy, thanks to the healthy fats found in good-quality bacon grease, butter, cream, and ranch dressing. This is the perfect soup to make when you want to use up some leftover chicken breast, but if you are using fresh chicken, simply roast it in the oven and shred with a fork to stir into your soup.

- 8 **bacon strips**
- 4 **tablespoons (60 g) butter**
- 1 **medium (150 g) yellow onion, chopped**
- 3 **garlic cloves, minced**
- 1 **teaspoon (5 g) sea salt**
- ½ **teaspoon (1 g) black pepper**
- 4 **cups (960 mL) chicken broth**
- 1 **cup (240 mL) heavy cream**
- 4 **tablespoons (60 g) cream cheese**
- ¼ **cup (60 mL) ranch dressing**
- 1 **pound (454 g) shredded cooked chicken breast**

INSTRUCTIONS:

Cook the bacon in a Dutch oven over medium heat until crispy, 5–7 minutes. Transfer the bacon to a plate. When cool enough to handle, crumble the bacon.

Pour off all but 2 tablespoons of bacon grease from the Dutch oven. Add the butter and melt over medium-low heat. Add the onion and garlic and sauté until soft, about 5 minutes. Season with the sea salt and black pepper and stir well to combine.

Add the chicken broth, cream, cream cheese, and ranch dressing, stir well, and bring to a simmer. Stir in the chicken and continue to simmer for 15 minutes.

Ladle the soup into bowls and garnish each serving with crumbled bacon. Store leftovers in an airtight container in the fridge for up to 3 days.

SERVES 4
PREP TIME: 15 MINUTES
COOKING TIME: 25 MINUTES

CALORIES: 726
CARBS: 6
PROTEIN: 44
FAT: 61

DAIRY-FREE CREAMY CHICKEN SOUP

Not everyone tolerates dairy well, so here is a recipe for those who need to omit it, or for those who simply want to try out another delicious keto recipe, filled with healthy fats and protein. Enjoy!

- **8 bacon strips**
- **1 medium (150 g) yellow onion, chopped**
- **3 garlic cloves, minced**
- **1 teaspoon (5 g) sea salt**
- **½ teaspoon (1 g) black pepper**
- **4 cups (400 g) cauliflower florets**
- **4 cups (960 mL) chicken broth**
- **1 cup (240 mL) canned coconut cream**
- **1 pound (454 g) boneless, skinless chicken breasts, cut into bite-size pieces**
- **Chopped fresh parsley, for garnish**

INSTRUCTIONS:

Cook the bacon in a Dutch oven over medium heat until crispy, 5–7 minutes. Transfer the bacon to a plate. When cool enough to handle, crumble the bacon.

Pour off all but 2 tablespoons of bacon grease from the Dutch oven and heat over medium-low heat. Add the onion and garlic and sauté until soft, about 5 minutes. Season with the sea salt and black pepper and stir well to combine. Add the cauliflower florets, chicken broth, and coconut cream and bring to a simmer. Stir in the chicken and continue to simmer for 15 minutes.

Ladle the soup into bowls and garnish each serving with crumbled bacon and parsley. Store leftovers in an airtight container in the fridge for up to 3 days.

SERVES 4

PREP TIME: 15 MINUTES

COOKING TIME: 25 MINUTES

CALORIES: 552

CARBS: 11

PROTEIN: 47

FAT: 37

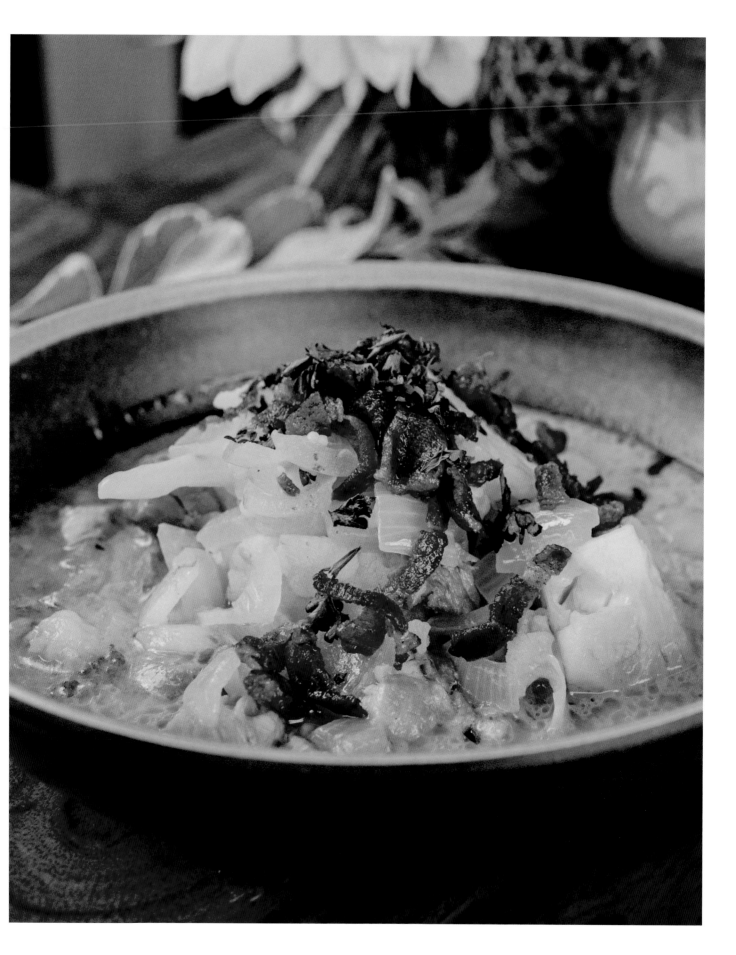

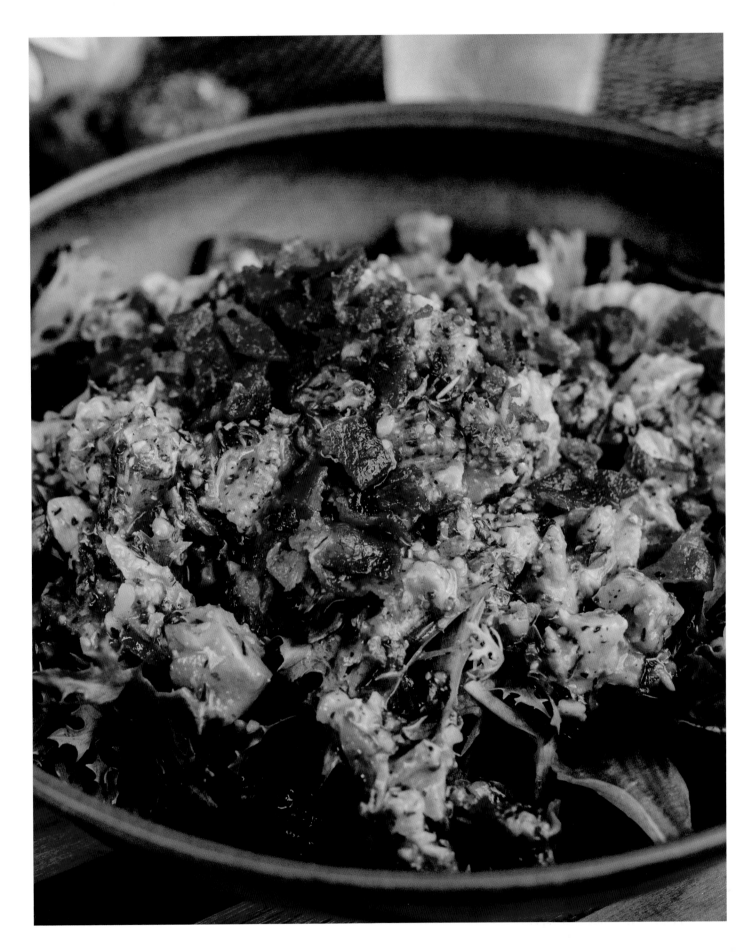

ITALIAN CHICKEN SALAD

Perfect for using up leftover chicken breast, this salad tastes amazing on its own or served alongside riced cauliflower and roasted sweet potatoes. You can increase the fat by adding some good-quality cheese.

- 2 **bacon strips**
- 6 **tablespoons (90 g) extra-virgin olive oil**
- 2 **tablespoons (30 mL) red wine vinegar**
- 1 **teaspoon (5 g) Dijon or stone-ground mustard**
- 1 **garlic clove, minced**
- 1 **scallion, minced**
- ½ **cup (32 g) minced fresh parsley**
- 1 **teaspoon (5 g) sea salt**
- ½ **teaspoon (1 g) black pepper**
- 1 **teaspoon (5 g) dried Italian seasoning**
- 1 **pound (454 g) cubed cooked chicken breast**
- 1 **medium (150 g) red bell pepper, seeded and chopped**
- **Mixed greens, for serving**

INSTRUCTIONS:

Cook the bacon in a skillet over medium heat until crispy, 5–7 minutes. Transfer the bacon to a plate. When cool enough to handle, crumble the bacon.

In a large bowl, combine the olive oil, vinegar, mustard, garlic, scallion, parsley, sea salt, black pepper, and Italian seasoning and whisk to mix well. Gently add the chicken, bell pepper, and bacon and toss to coat.

Serve on a bed of mixed greens. Store leftovers in an airtight container in the fridge for up to 3 days.

SERVES 4
PREP TIME: 15 MINUTES
COOKING TIME: 5 MINUTES

CALORIES: 398
CARBS: 2
PROTEIN: 37
FAT: 26

GREEK YOGURT CHICKEN SALAD

This salad is ultra-creamy, thanks to full-fat Greek yogurt and mayonnaise as its base. Opt for the highest quality you can find: yogurt without additives and mayonnaise without inflammatory oils and sugar.

GREEK YOGURT DRESSING:

- 7 ounces (200 g) full-fat Greek yogurt
- ¼ cup (60 g) mayonnaise
- 2 tablespoons (30 g) yellow mustard
- 1 scallion, minced
- ½ cup (32 g) minced fresh parsley
- Grated zest of ½ lemon
- 1 teaspoon (5 g) sea salt
- ½ teaspoon (1 g) black pepper

CHICKEN SALAD:

- 4 medium (200 g) celery stalks, diced
- 1 medium (200 g) cucumber, diced
- 1 cup (150 g) cherry tomatoes, halved
- 8 ounces (228 g) shredded cooked chicken breast
- 1 medium (150 g) avocado, peeled, pitted, and diced

INSTRUCTIONS:

Whisk together all the dressing ingredients in a large bowl.

Add all the salad ingredients to the bowl and gently toss until everything is coated in the dressing.

Serve. Store leftovers in an airtight container in the fridge for up to 3 days.

SERVES 4
PREP TIME: 15 MINUTES

CALORIES: 327
CARBS: 9
PROTEIN: 25
FAT: 22

SLOW COOKER CHICKEN ALFREDO

Using your slow cooker for this recipe saves time and energy and will leave your home smelling like nourishing comfort as this creamy chicken alfredo simmers and its flavors meld together.

2 cups (480 mL) heavy cream

1 cup (240 mL) chicken broth

1 teaspoon (5 g) sea salt

½ teaspoon (1 g) black pepper

1 teaspoon (5 g) red pepper flakes

Pinch ground nutmeg

2 tablespoons (30 g) butter

1 pound (454 g) boneless, skinless chicken breasts, cut into bite-size pieces

3 garlic cloves, minced

4 cups (288 g) broccoli florets

1 cup (100 g) shredded Parmesan cheese

INSTRUCTIONS:

Combine the cream, chicken broth, sea salt, black pepper, red pepper flakes, and nutmeg in a slow cooker and whisk well. Add the butter, chicken, garlic, and broccoli florets and gently toss in the cream mixture.

Cover and cook on low for 4 hours or on high for 3 hours. Stir in the Parmesan cheese and serve.

Store leftovers in an airtight container in the fridge for up to 3 days.

SERVES 4

PREP TIME: 10 MINUTES

COOKING TIME: 3–4 HOURS

CALORIES: 698

CARBS: 9

PROTEIN: 35

FAT: 62

CREAM CHEESE TURKEY SOUP

We know you will love this extra-creamy soup as much as we do! If you don't have a slow cooker, you can simmer this soup in a large pot on the stove for 30–40 minutes, until the veggies are very soft and everything is bubbling together.

- 2 **tablespoons (30 g) butter**
- 1 **medium (150 g) yellow onion, diced**
- 3 **garlic cloves, diced**
- 1 **teaspoon (5 g) sea salt**
- ½ **teaspoon (1 g) black pepper**
- ½ **teaspoon (2.5 g) red pepper flakes**
- 2 **cups (200 g) cremini mushrooms, sliced**
- 1 **pound (454 g) shredded cooked turkey**
- 2 **cups (480 mL) chicken stock or bone broth**
- 1 **cup (240 mL) heavy cream**
- 8 **ounces (228 g) cream cheese**
- 1 **cup (114 g) shredded Cheddar cheese**

Minced fresh parsley and/ or cilantro, for garnish

INSTRUCTIONS:

Melt the butter in a large skillet over medium heat. Add the onion and garlic and sauté until soft, about 5 minutes. Season with the sea salt, black pepper, and red pepper flakes. Add the mushrooms and sauté until soft, about 3 minutes.

Transfer the mixture to a slow cooker. Add the turkey, broth, cream, cream cheese, and shredded cheese, cover, and cook on low for 4 hours or on high for 3 hours.

Serve, garnished with fresh parsley or cilantro, or both!

SERVES 4
PREP TIME: 15 MINUTES
COOKING TIME: 3–4 HOURS

CALORIES: 684
CARBS: 16
PROTEIN: 47
FAT: 47

CHEESY FRENCH ONION CHICKEN CASSEROLE

We took the classic flavors of French onion soup and used them in this baked casserole dish, featuring chicken instead of bread. Opting for protein instead of carbs will keep you fuller longer and feeling better overall. Serve this with your favorite roasted veggies, sweet potatoes, or a big salad and enjoy!

- 2 **tablespoons (30 g) butter**
- 2 **medium (150 g) yellow onions, diced**
- 1 **teaspoon (5 g) sea salt**
- ½ **teaspoon (1 g) black pepper**
- ½ **cup (120 mL) chicken stock or bone broth**
- 2 **garlic cloves, minced**
- 1 **pound (454 g) boneless, skinless chicken breasts**
- 1 **teaspoon (5 g) dried oregano**
- 1 **teaspoon (5 g) red pepper flakes**
- 1 **cup (114 g) shredded Gruyère cheese**
- 1 **cup (114 g) shredded mozzarella cheese**
- **Minced fresh parsley, for garnish**

INSTRUCTIONS:

Preheat the oven to 400°F (200°C). Butter a large baking dish and set aside.

Melt the butter in a large skillet over medium-high heat. Add the onions, season with the sea salt and black pepper, and sauté until soft, about 5 minutes. Reduce the heat to medium-low and continue to cook, stirring occasionally, until the onions are very soft and have caramelized (turned brown), about 15 minutes. Pour in the chicken stock, scraping any browned bits of onion. Add the garlic and cook until fragrant, about 1 minute. Remove the skillet from the heat and set aside.

Place the chicken breasts in a single layer in the prepared baking dish and season with the oregano and red pepper flakes. Scatter the caramelized onions evenly on top of each chicken breast. Sprinkle the shredded cheeses on top. Bake until the chicken is cooked through (165°F/75°C) and the cheese is bubbly, 20–25 minutes.

Switch the oven to broil. Place the baking dish under the broiler until browned, about 2 minutes. Garnish with fresh parsley and serve.

SERVES 4
PREP TIME: 15 MINUTES
COOKING TIME: 50 MINUTES

CALORIES: 452
CARBS: 6
PROTEIN: 44
FAT: 28

CHICKEN WITH ROASTED PEPPERS AND PARMESAN

Just toss the ingredients into a cast-iron skillet and put it in the oven, and you'll have a warm and comforting dinner in no time! Serve on its own or over a bed of riced cauliflower or roasted butternut squash.

- 1 **pound (454 g) bone-in, skin-on chicken thighs**
- 2 **medium (150 g) red bell peppers, seeded and diced**
- 20 **cherry tomatoes**
- 2 **garlic cloves, minced**
- 6 **tablespoons (90 g) butter, cut into small pieces**
- 1 **tablespoon (15 mL) red wine vinegar**
- 1 **teaspoon (5 g) sea salt**
- ½ **teaspoon (1 g) black pepper**
- 1 **teaspoon (5 g) smoked paprika**

  Pinch cayenne pepper
- 1 **cup (100 g) grated Parmesan cheese**

  Minced fresh basil, for garnish

INSTRUCTIONS:

Preheat the oven to 350°F (180°C).

Place the chicken thighs in a single layer in an 8-inch cast-iron skillet. Scatter the bell peppers, cherry tomatoes, and garlic around the chicken. Sprinkle the butter pieces and vinegar over the entire dish, season with the sea salt, black pepper, smoked paprika, and cayenne, and sprinkle the Parmesan cheese over everything.

Bake until the chicken is cooked through (165°F/75°C) and the chicken skin and Parmesan cheese are golden, about 35 minutes. Garnish with the basil and serve.

SERVES 4

PREP TIME: 15 MINUTES

COOKING TIME: 35 MINUTES

CALORIES: 557

CARBS: 9

PROTEIN: 29

FAT: 44

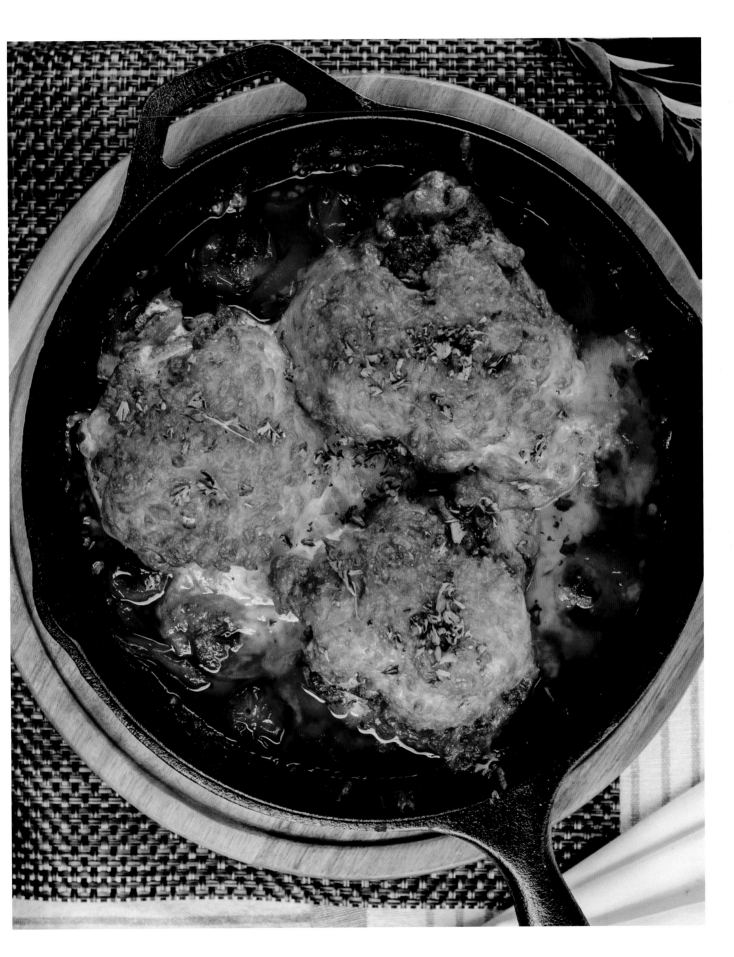

GARLIC BUTTER CHICKEN THIGHS AND GREEN BEANS

Mixing butter with coconut aminos, fresh garlic, spices, and lemon zest creates a delicious, mouthwatering flavor punch on top of bone-in chicken thighs and French green beans. Serve wedges of fresh lemon for squeezing.

- 1 **pound (454 g) bone-in, skin-on chicken thighs**
- 4 **cups (600 g) French green beans**
- 6 **tablespoons (90 g) butter**
- 2 **tablespoons (30 mL) coconut aminos**
- 2 **garlic cloves, peeled**

  Grated zest of ½ lemon
- 1 **teaspoon (5 g) smoked paprika**
- 1 **teaspoon (5 g) sea salt**
- ½ **teaspoon (1 g) black pepper**

  Minced fresh parsley, for garnish

INSTRUCTIONS:

Preheat the oven to 350°F (180°C).

Place the chicken thighs in a single layer in a baking dish. Scatter the green beans around the chicken thighs.

Combine the butter, coconut aminos, garlic, lemon zest, smoked paprika, sea salt, and black pepper in a food processor and process until creamy. Dollop the butter mixture over each piece of chicken.

Bake until the chicken is cooked through (165°F/75°C) and the skin is golden, about 35 minutes. Garnish with fresh parsley and serve.

SERVES 4
PREP TIME: 15 MINUTES
COOKING TIME: 35 MINUTES

CALORIES: 433
CARBS: 5
PROTEIN: 28
FAT: 34

SPINACH AND CHICKEN CASSEROLE

This comforting dish will be one of your favorites, as it combines familiar flavors from cheese and spices and smothers it all over chicken thighs—yum!

- 1 **pound (454 g) boneless, skinless chicken thighs**
- 4 **cups (120 g) baby spinach, chopped**
- 8 **ounces (228 g) cream cheese**
- 4 **tablespoons (60 g) butter, cut into small pieces**
- 2 **garlic cloves, peeled**
- 1 **teaspoon (5 g) sea salt**
- ½ **teaspoon (1 g) black pepper**
- 1 **teaspoon (5 g) Italian seasoning**
- **Pinch ground nutmeg**
- 1 **cup (228 g) shredded mozzarella cheese**
- **Grated zest of ½ lemon**
- **Minced fresh parsley, for garnish**

INSTRUCTIONS:

Preheat the oven to 400°F (200°C).

Place the chicken thighs in a single layer in a baking dish.

Mix the baby spinach, cream cheese, butter, garlic, sea salt, black pepper, Italian seasoning, nutmeg, shredded mozzarella, and lemon zest in a food processor until creamy. Spread the cheese mixture over each chicken thigh.

Bake until the chicken is cooked through (165°F/75°C) and the cheese mixture is bubbly, about 30 minutes.

Garnish with fresh parsley and serve.

SERVES 4
PREP TIME: 15 MINUTES
COOKING TIME: 30 MINUTES

CALORIES: 499
CARBS: 6
PROTEIN: 30
FAT: 38

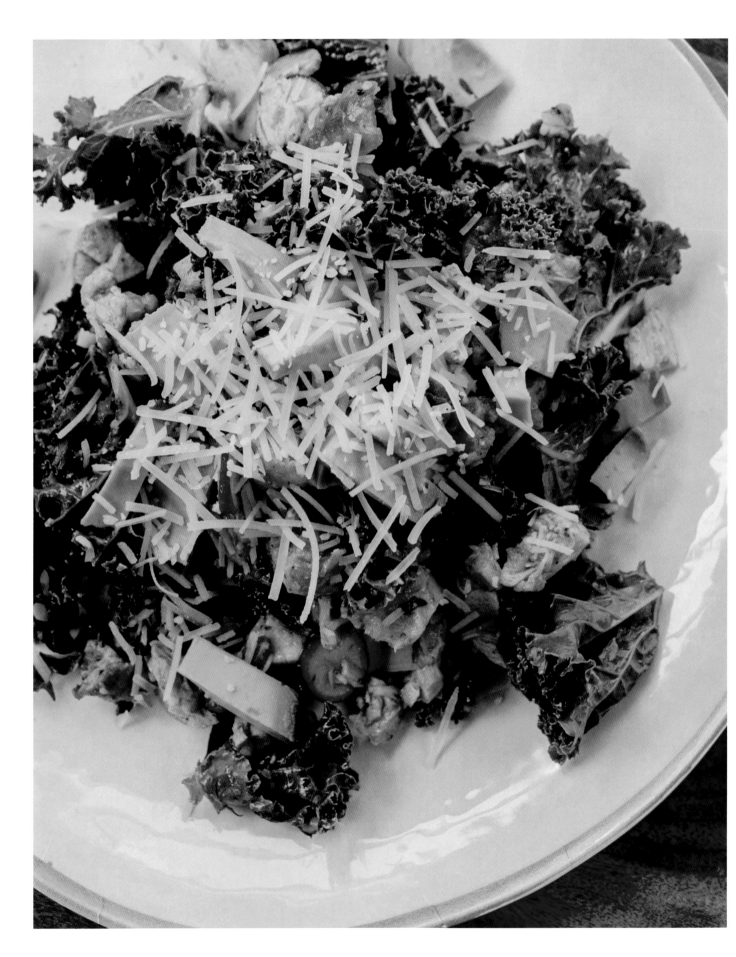

LEMON-BASIL CHICKEN SALAD

A fresh green salad made with leftover chicken is just the ticket on a warm day after work, so get this on your menu to make soon! Creamy avocado pairs perfectly with crunchy radish, all coated in a bright lemon-basil vinaigrette.

VINAIGRETTE:

- ¼ cup (60 mL) extra-virgin olive oil
- 2 tablespoons (30 mL) fresh lemon juice
- 1 tablespoon (15 mL) red wine vinegar
- 1 scallion, minced
- 10 fresh basil leaves, chopped
- 1 teaspoon (5 g) sea salt
- ½ teaspoon (1 g) black pepper
- 1 teaspoon (5 g) red pepper flakes
- 1 teaspoon (5 g) Italian seasoning

SALAD:

- 6 cups (255 g) baby kale
- 8 ounces (228 g) cooked chicken thighs, cut into bite-size pieces
- 4 radishes, trimmed and thinly sliced
- Grated zest of ½ lemon
- 1 medium (150 g) avocado, peeled, pitted, and diced

GARNISH:

- ½ cup (50 g) shredded Parmesan cheese

INSTRUCTIONS:

Blend all the vinaigrette ingredients together in a food processor or blender until creamy. Pour into a large bowl. Add all the salad ingredients to the bowl and gently toss until everything is coated in the vinaigrette. Sprinkle the Parmesan cheese on top and serve.

SERVES 2
PREP TIME: 15 MINUTES

CALORIES: 655
CARBS: 10
PROTEIN: 46
FAT: 47

CHICKEN NOODLE SOUP

What's better than a warm bowl of chicken noodle soup on a day when you need a bit of extra comfort? We love how versatile zucchini noodles are, so we added them to our favorite soup. You're going to love this.

- 2 tablespoons (30 g) butter
- 1 medium (150 g) yellow onion, minced
- 2 garlic cloves, minced
- 4 medium (200 g) celery stalks, diced
- 2 medium (100 g) carrots, peeled and diced
- 1 pound (454 g) boneless, skinless chicken thighs, cut into bite-size pieces
- 2 cups (250 g) zucchini noodles
- 1 scallion, minced
- 1 teaspoon (5 g) sea salt
- ½ teaspoon (1 g) black pepper
- 1 teaspoon (5 g) red pepper flakes
- 1 teaspoon (5 g) Italian seasoning
- 4 cups (960 mL) chicken stock or bone broth
- Grated zest of ½ lemon
- ¼ cup (16 g) minced fresh parsley
- 1 medium (150 g) avocado, peeled, pitted, and diced
- ½ cup (50 g) grated Parmesan cheese, for garnish

INSTRUCTIONS:

Melt the butter in a large skillet over medium-low heat. Add the onion and garlic and sauté until soft, about 5 minutes. Add the celery and carrots and continue to sauté until soft, about 5 minutes. Add the chicken and cook, until it browns a bit, stirring often, about 5 minutes. Stir in the zucchini noodles and scallion and season with the sea salt, black pepper, red pepper flakes, and Italian seasoning.

Pour in the chicken stock, bring to a simmer, and cook until all the veggies are soft and the chicken is cooked through, about 10 minutes.

Turn off the heat and stir in the lemon zest, parsley, and diced avocado. Ladle the soup into bowls and garnish each serving with a sprinkle of grated Parmesan cheese.

SERVES 4
PREP TIME: 15 MINUTES
COOKING TIME: 25 MINUTES

CALORIES: 409
CARBS: 12
PROTEIN: 36
FAT: 27

TURKEY AND BELL PEPPER SKILLET

This dish is rich in flavor and healthy fats, sure to leave you feeling satisfied and grounded in your body. A sprinkle of grated cheese on top would be a nice addition, but it's perfect just as given here.

2 tablespoons (30 g) butter, divided

1 pound (454 g) turkey tenderloin

1 teaspoon (5 g) sea salt

½ teaspoon (1 g) black pepper

1 medium (150 g) yellow onion, sliced

2 garlic cloves, minced

2 teaspoons (10 g) chili powder

2 medium (150 g) bell peppers (any color), seeded and sliced

10 cherry tomatoes, halved

1 tablespoon (15 mL) red wine vinegar

GARNISH:

Minced fresh cilantro

1 **medium (150 g) avocado, peeled, pitted, and diced**

¼ **cup (60 mL) extra-virgin olive oil**

¼ **cup (60 g) full-fat sour cream**

INSTRUCTIONS:

Melt 1 tablespoon of the butter in a cast-iron skillet over medium heat. Add the turkey, season with the sea salt and black pepper, and cook until browned, about 3 minutes per side. Transfer the turkey to a plate.

Add the remaining 1 tablespoon butter to the skillet. When melted, add the onion and garlic and sauté until soft, about 5 minutes, scraping up all the browned bits in the skillet. Sprinkle with the chili powder. Add the bell peppers, cherry tomatoes, and red wine vinegar and continue to sauté until soft, about 5 minutes.

Serve the turkey and veggies garnished with fresh cilantro, avocado, a drizzle of olive oil, and a dollop of sour cream.

SERVES 4
PREP TIME: 15 MINUTES
COOKING TIME: 20 MINUTES

CALORIES: 431
CARBS: 10
PROTEIN: 31
FAT: 28

MUSTARD CHICKEN STIR-FRY

This dish combines the bright and tangy flavor of mustard with the velvety fattiness of bacon, so we don't know how you wouldn't love it! We kept the fat content higher in this recipe by using chicken thighs instead of breast.

- ¼ cup (60 mL) extra-virgin olive oil
- 2 tablespoons (30 mL) fresh lemon juice
- ½ cup (50 g) grated Parmesan cheese
- ¼ cup (60 g) yellow or stone-ground mustard
- 1 teaspoon (5 g) sea salt
- 1 pound (454 g) boneless, skinless chicken thighs, cut into bite-size pieces
- 2 bacon strips
- 1 tablespoon (15 g) butter
- 1 medium (150 g) yellow onion, minced
- 2 garlic cloves, minced
- 2 cups (200 g) cauliflower florets
- 1 medium (150 g) yellow or green bell pepper, seeded and sliced

GARNISH:

- Chopped fresh parsley
  Toasted sesame seeds

INSTRUCTIONS:

Combine the olive oil, lemon juice, Parmesan cheese, mustard, and sea salt in a large bowl, add the chicken, and toss to coat well. Cover and marinate the chicken in the fridge for at least 2 hours or up to overnight.

Cook the bacon in a skillet over medium heat until crispy, 5–7 minutes. Transfer the bacon to a plate. When cool enough to handle, crumble the bacon. Pour off most of the bacon grease from the skillet, reserving 2 tablespoons for serving.

Melt the butter in the same skillet. Add the chicken, onion, and garlic and sauté until the chicken is cooked through, about 10 minutes. Add the cauliflower florets and bell pepper, toss well, and sauté until the cauliflower is soft, about 5 minutes.

Serve the chicken and veggies topped with crumbled bacon, parsley, sesame seeds, and a drizzle of bacon grease.

SERVES 4

PREP TIME: 15 MINUTES, PLUS 2 HOURS TO MARINATE

COOKING TIME: 20 MINUTES

CALORIES: 367

CARBS: 11

PROTEIN: 23

FAT: 26

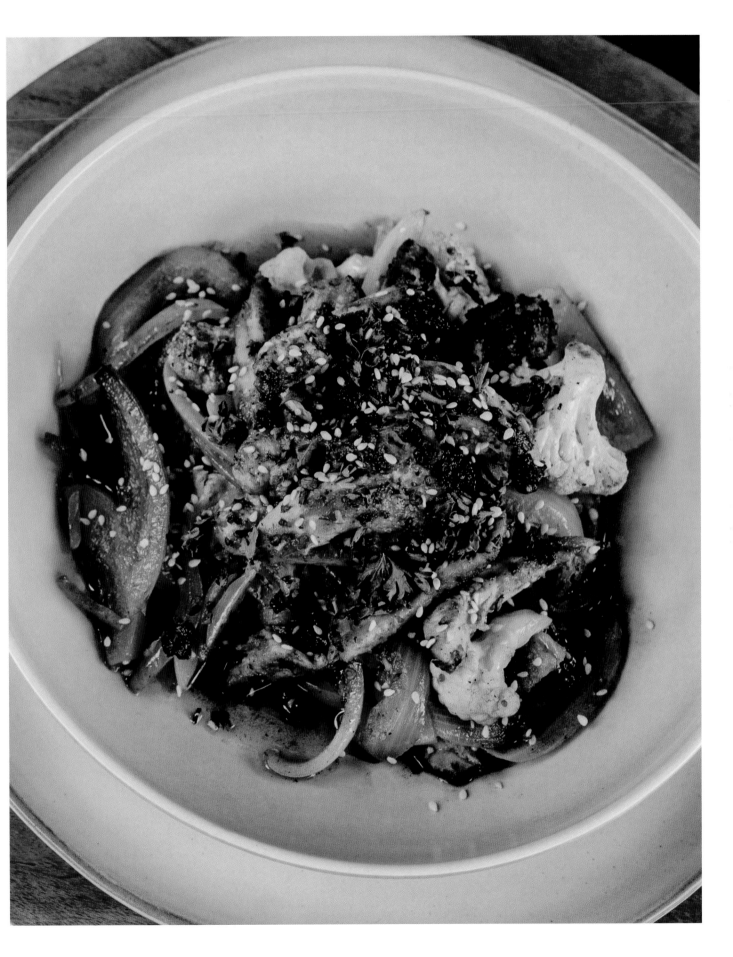

CHICKEN AND CAULIFLOWER IN CREAMY WHITE WINE SAUCE

A skillet meal is just perfect for dinner tonight with this fast and easy recipe. Let the flavors from this dish meld together to create something truly special and delicious!

CAULIFLOWER:

- **2 tablespoons (30 g) butter**
- **2 cups (500 g) riced cauliflower**
- **1 teaspoon (5 g) sea salt**

CHICKEN:

- **1 pound (454 g) chicken tenders**
- **Sea salt, black pepper, and garlic powder to taste**

SAUCE:

- **4 tablespoons (60 g) butter**
- **1 cup (240 mL) heavy cream**
- **½ cup (120 mL) dry white wine**
- **1 tablespoon (15 mL) fresh lemon juice**
- **2 garlic cloves, minced**
- **1 teaspoon (5 g) sea salt**
- **½ teaspoon (1 g) black pepper**
- **1 teaspoon (5 g) dried thyme**

GARNISH:

- **Minced fresh parsley**

INSTRUCTIONS:

Melt the butter in a cast-iron skillet over medium heat. Add the riced cauliflower and sea salt and cook, stirring often, until softened, about 3 minutes. Transfer the riced cauliflower to a serving dish.

Add the chicken tenders to the skillet and sprinkle with sea salt, black pepper, and garlic powder. Sear the chicken without stirring until well browned, 4–6 minutes per side. Add the chicken to the dish with the riced cauliflower.

To make the sauce, melt the butter in the same skillet. Add the cream, wine, lemon juice, garlic, sea salt, black pepper, and thyme and bring to a simmer, scraping up the bits of browned chicken. Cook, stirring often, until the sauce has thickened, about 10 minutes.

Pour the sauce over the riced cauliflower and chicken, garnish with fresh parsley, and serve.

SERVES 4
PREP TIME: 5 MINUTES
COOKING TIME: 20 MINUTES

CALORIES: 515
CARBS: 8
PROTEIN: 27
FAT: 38

CILANTRO-PECAN PESTO CHICKEN

We put an unexpected twist on traditional pesto by adding some fresh cilantro and chopped pecans along with a few cherry tomatoes, then served it over sautéed ground chicken. Dig in—we know you're going to love it!

CILANTRO-PECAN PESTO:

- ¼ **cup (60 mL) extra-virgin olive oil**
- 2 **cups (32 g) fresh cilantro leaves**
- 2 **cups (40 g) fresh basil leaves**
- 1 **garlic clove, peeled**
- 1 **teaspoon (5 g) sea salt**
- ¼ **cup (28 g) chopped pecans**
- 2 **tablespoons (30 mL) fresh lemon juice**
- ½ **cup (50 g) grated Parmesan cheese**
- 5 **cherry tomatoes**

CHICKEN:

- 1 **tablespoon (15 g) butter**
- 1 **pound (454 g) ground chicken**
- 1 **medium (150 g) yellow onion, minced**
- 3 **garlic cloves, minced**
- 2 **teaspoons (10 g) sea salt**
- 1 **teaspoon (2 g) black pepper**
- 1 **teaspoon (5 g) red pepper flakes**

INSTRUCTIONS:

Combine all the pesto ingredients in a high-speed blender or food processor and blend until creamy. Set aside until ready to use.

Melt the butter in a large skillet over medium-high heat. Add the ground chicken, onion, and garlic and cook until the chicken is cooked through and crumbly, 5–7 minutes.

Season the chicken with the sea salt, black pepper, and red pepper flakes. Pour the pesto over the cooked chicken in the skillet and toss until the chicken is coated.

SERVES 4
PREP TIME: 10 MINUTES
COOKING TIME: 10 MINUTES

CALORIES: 463
CARBS: 11
PROTEIN: 26
FAT: 35

TURKEY AND BUTTERNUT GOULASH

This warm autumn dish is just the ticket for the cooler, shorter days. We top ours with creamy avocado and sour cream to ensure it has enough healthy fats to help us feel grounded and satisfied.

- 2 tablespoons (30 g) butter
- 1 pound (454 g) ground turkey
- 1 medium (150 g) yellow onion, diced
- 3 garlic cloves, minced
- 4 cups (560 g) cubed butternut squash
- 2 teaspoons (10 g) sea salt
- 1 teaspoon (2 g) black pepper
- 1 teaspoon (5 g) red pepper flakes
- 1 tablespoon (15 g) smoked paprika
- 2 cups (480 mL) chicken stock

GARNISH:

- 1 medium (150 g) avocado, peeled, pitted, and diced
- 1 scallion, minced

Minced fresh cilantro

INSTRUCTIONS:

Melt the butter in a stockpot over medium heat. Add the turkey and cook until the turkey has browned, 5–7 minutes. Add the onion and garlic and cook, stirring often, until transparent, about 5 minutes. Add the butternut squash, sea salt, black pepper, red pepper flakes, and smoked paprika. Cook, stirring frequently, until fragrant, about 2 minutes. Add the chicken stock and bring to a simmer. Cook until thickened to the desired consistency, 20–30 minutes.

Serve topped with avocado, scallion, and cilantro.

SERVES 4
PREP TIME: 15 MINUTES
COOKING TIME: 30 MINUTES

CALORIES: 370
CARBS: 15
PROTEIN: 20
FAT: 27

CHICKEN AND BROCCOLI CASSEROLE

Crushed pork rinds give this dish an extra-salty texture that you and your family will love. We used Cheddar cheese in this dish, but you could also use Monterey Jack, Colby, or mozzarella!

- 2 **cups (156 g) broccoli florets**
- 1 **tablespoon (15 mL) extra-virgin olive oil**
- 1 **pound (454 g) shredded cooked chicken breast**
- 3 **garlic cloves, minced**
- 2 **tablespoons (30 g) butter**
- ½ **cup (114 g) heavy cream**
- 4 **ounces (114 g) cream cheese, cut into small pieces**
- 2 **cups (228 g) shredded Cheddar cheese**
- 2 **teaspoons (10 g) sea salt**
- 1 **teaspoon (2 g) black pepper**
- 1 **teaspoon (5 g) red pepper flakes**
- **Pinch ground nutmeg**
- 2 **cups (70 g) crushed pork rinds**

INSTRUCTIONS:

Preheat the oven to 350°F (180°C).

Pour an inch or two of water into a small saucepan with a steamer basket insert. Cover and bring to a boil over medium-high heat. Add the broccoli florets to the steamer basket, cover, and steam until tender, about 6 minutes. Drain.

Pour the olive oil into a 9 × 13-inch baking dish and spread it all over the bottom and sides. Place the cooked chicken in a single layer in the bottom of the dish. Scatter the steamed broccoli evenly over the chicken and scatter the minced garlic over it all.

Melt the butter in a saucepan over medium heat. Add the cream and cook, stirring often, for 2 minutes. Stir in the cream cheese pieces until melted and smooth, 2–3 minutes. Add the Cheddar cheese and stir until melted, 2–3 minutes. Season with the sea salt, black pepper, red pepper flakes, and nutmeg. Pour the sauce over the chicken and broccoli and top with the crushed pork rinds.

Bake until the sauce is bubbly, 30–35 minutes.

SERVES 6
PREP TIME: 15 MINUTES
COOKING TIME: 45 MINUTES

CALORIES: 406
CARBS: 6
PROTEIN: 44
FAT: 54

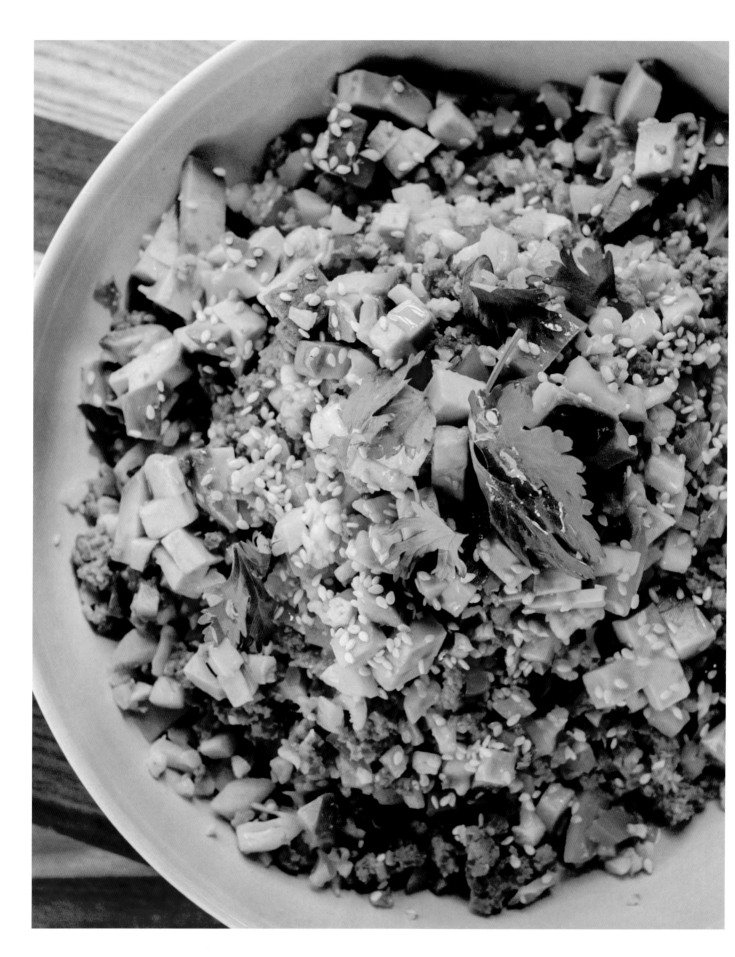

TURKEY TERIYAKI RICE BOWLS

These rice bowls will become one of your family's favorites, and they don't take long to prepare at all! Let everyone add their own garnishes to make this meal a family event.

- 1 tablespoon (15 mL) extra-virgin olive oil
- 1 pound (454 g) ground turkey
- 1 medium (150 g) yellow onion, diced
- 3 garlic cloves, minced
- 1 medium (150 g) red or yellow bell pepper, seeded and diced
- 1 teaspoon (5 g) sea salt
- 1 teaspoon (5 g) red pepper flakes
- 1 tablespoon (15 mL) fresh lime juice
- 2 tablespoons (30 mL) coconut aminos
- 4 cups (1000 g) riced cauliflower
- 1 scallion, minced

GARNISH:

- ¼ cup (60 mL) toasted sesame seed oil
- 1 medium (150 g) avocado, peeled, pitted, and diced
- Minced fresh cilantro
- 1 tablespoon (15 g) sesame seeds

INSTRUCTIONS:

In a large skillet, heat the oil over medium-high heat. Add the ground turkey and cook, crumbling the meat while cooking, until it begins to brown, about 5 minutes. Add the onion, garlic, and bell pepper and cook until the turkey is well browned and the vegetables are soft, about 6 minutes, stirring occasionally to prevent burning.

Season with the sea salt, red pepper flakes, lime juice, and coconut aminos and stir to mix well. Add the riced cauliflower and scallion and cook until softened, stirring often, about 5 minutes.

Serve topped with toasted sesame seed oil, diced avocado, fresh cilantro, and sesame seeds.

SERVES 4
PREP TIME: 5 MINUTES
COOKING TIME: 15 MINUTES

CALORIES: 486
CARBS: 14
PROTEIN: 25
FAT: 35

SHEET PAN SRIRACHA CHICKEN THIGHS

This sheet pan meal will have your dinner on the table in no time, with little cleanup to follow. If you don't have sriracha sauce, any chili-garlic or hot sauce will do.

MARINADE:

- 2 tablespoons (30 mL) sriracha sauce
- ¼ cup (60 mL) toasted sesame oil
- 1 tablespoon (15 mL) coconut aminos
- 1 tablespoon (15 mL) rice vinegar
- 2 garlic cloves, minced
- 2 teaspoons (10 g) sea salt
- 1 teaspoon (2 g) black pepper

CHICKEN AND VEGGIES:

- 4 (6-ounce/684 g) bone-in, skin-on chicken thighs
- 2 cups (200 g) cauliflower florets
- 1 medium (150 g) red bell pepper, seeded and sliced
- Minced fresh parsley, for garnish

INSTRUCTIONS:

Preheat the oven to 400°F (200°C).

Mix together all the marinade ingredients in a baking dish. Add the chicken thighs, cauliflower florets, and red bell pepper slices and gently toss to coat. Bake until the chicken reaches 165°F (75°C), 35–40 minutes.

Serve topped with parsley.

SERVES 4
PREP TIME: 10 MINUTES
COOKING TIME: 40 MINUTES

CALORIES: 599
CARBS: 6
PROTEIN: 30
FAT: 49

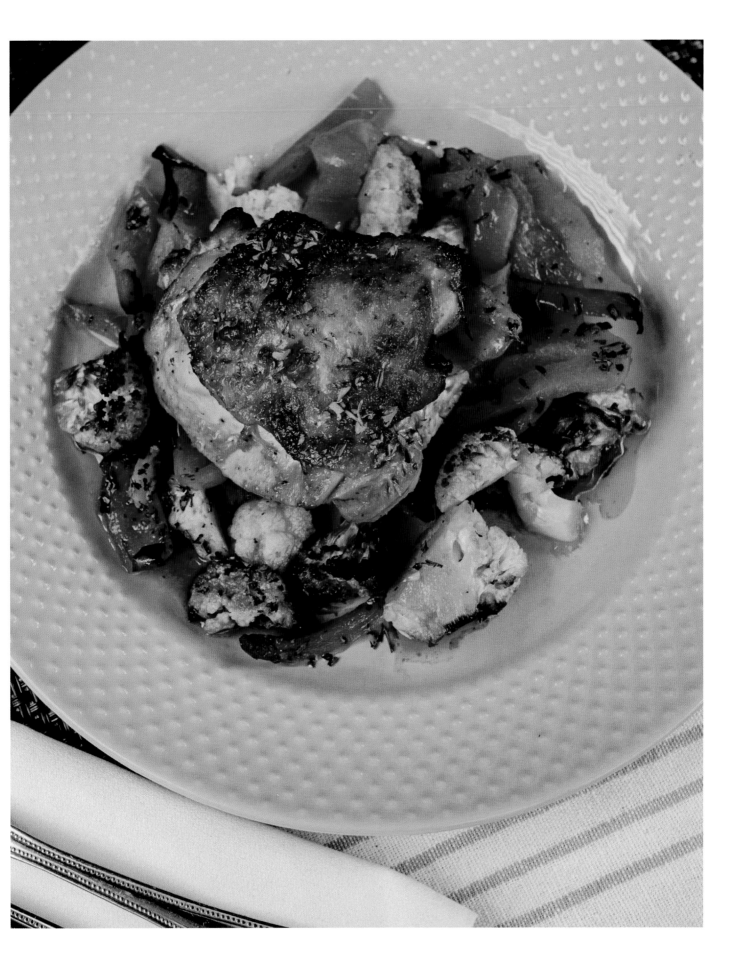

MEAT
ENTREES

CHAPTER 7

Fire up your grill, get out your cast-iron skillet, or use your pressure cooker for these tasty recipes featuring grass-fed beef, pasture-raised fowl, and heritage breed pork. These recipes range from simple preparations with minimal ingredients to more exotic gourmet recipes for those special occasions when you have more time and energy. When you source the most sustainably raised meats, you boost nutritional value and minimize moral and environmental objections to eating meat.

PRESSURE-COOKED PORK SHOULDER

An Instant Pot electric pressure cooker is perfect for this recipe, as you'll have melt-in-your-mouth pork shoulder that tastes like it's been slow-cooking all day in just a couple of hours.

- 1 tablespoon (15 g) ghee or butter
- 3½ pounds (1596 g) boneless pork shoulder (do not remove twine)
- 1 cup (240 mL) beef or chicken bone broth
- 1 medium (150 g) yellow onion, minced
- 2 medium (100 g) carrots, peeled and chopped
- 4 medium (200 g) celery stalks, diced
- 2 cups (180 g) sliced cremini mushrooms
- 2 tablespoons (30 mL) raw apple cider vinegar
- 2 tablespoons (30 mL) coconut aminos
- ¼ cup (60 mL) keto-friendly BBQ sauce

- 2 teaspoons (10 g) sea salt
- 1 teaspoon (2 g) cracked black pepper
- 1 tablespoon (3.75 g) garlic powder
- 1 teaspoon (5 g) dried oregano
- 1 teaspoon (5 g) dried rosemary
- ½ cup (32 g) minced fresh parsley
- 2 scallions, minced

INSTRUCTIONS:

Melt the ghee in a large Dutch oven or stockpot over medium-high heat. Add the pork shoulder and brown all over, about 2 minutes per side.

Pour the bone broth into a pressure cooker. Add the seared pork shoulder, followed by the onion, carrots, celery, and mushrooms. Pour in the apple cider vinegar and coconut aminos. Pour the BBQ sauce over the pork shoulder and use your hands to carefully rub it into the pork. Season with the sea salt, black pepper, garlic powder, dried oregano, and dried rosemary.

Cook on the MEAT setting with the steam valve sealed for 1 hour, then allow the steam to release naturally for at least 20 minutes. Remove from pressure cooker and remove the twine. Top with the parsley and scallions and serve.

Store leftovers in an airtight container in the fridge for up to 3 days.

SERVES 8
PREP TIME: 20 MINUTES
COOKING TIME: 1½ HOURS

CALORIES: 469
CARBS: 7
PROTEIN: 41
FAT: 31

MEXICAN SALAD IN CHEDDAR CHEESE SHELLS

You won't be missing the corn tortillas in this recipe featuring Cheddar cheese taco shells! We fill them with spiced ground beef and lots of fresh veggies. Double the recipe to serve a crowd or for repeat servings during a busy week.

- 8 (1-ounce/28 g) slices Cheddar cheese
- 12 ounces (336 g) ground beef
- 2 tablespoons (30 g) keto-friendly (sugar-free) taco seasoning
- 2 teaspoons (10 g) sea salt
- 1 teaspoon (1.25 g) garlic powder
- 4 cups (170 g) baby kale, minced
- 20 cherry tomatoes, sliced in half
- 4 medium radishes, diced
- 1 medium (150 g) avocado, peeled, pitted, and diced
- 1½ ounces (43 g) crumbled feta cheese

INSTRUCTIONS:

Preheat the oven to 350°F (180°C). Line a rimmed baking sheet with parchment paper.

Place the slices of cheese in a single layer on the prepared baking sheet. Bake until completely melted and bubbling, about 7 minutes.

While the cheese is baking, cook the ground beef in a large skillet over medium heat, breaking up the meat, until browned, about 10 minutes. Season with the taco seasoning, sea salt, and garlic powder.

Remove the baking sheet from the oven and allow to cool for 2 minutes, then cut around each slice of cheese to make it easy to peel each slice off the parchment paper. Carefully stuff each cheese slice in the cup of a muffin tin to form a shell. Allow the cheese cups to cool and harden a bit, then stuff each cheese cup with the ground beef, kale, tomatoes, radishes, avocado, and feta. Store leftovers in the fridge for up to 3 days.

SERVES 4
PREP TIME: 10 MINUTES
COOKING TIME: 10 MINUTES

CALORIES: 573
CARBS: 10
PROTEIN: 37
FAT: 40

TRADITIONAL BEEF STEW

This traditional beef stew simmers slowly on the stovetop, warming up your kitchen with its hearty flavors. You'll be so excited to dig into this!

- 2 tablespoons (30 g) butter
- 2 cups (200 g) mushrooms, chopped
- 1¼ pounds (570 g) beef chuck roast, cubed
- 2 tablespoons (30 g) tomato paste
- 3 garlic cloves, minced
- 1 large bay leaf
- 1 teaspoon (5 g) dried thyme
- 4 cups (960 mL) beef broth, divided
- 1 medium (150 g) yellow onion, chopped
- 4 medium (200 g) celery stalks, chopped
- 2 medium (100 g) carrots, peeled and chopped
- 2 cups (300 g) cherry tomatoes, halved
- 1 teaspoon (5 g) sea salt
- ½ teaspoon (1 g) black pepper

INSTRUCTIONS:

Melt the butter in a Dutch oven or stock pot over medium heat. Add the mushrooms and stir to coat. Let sear for 2 minutes, then stir and cook for 2 minutes more. Transfer the mushrooms to a plate.

Brown the cubed beef in the pot in batches, adding more butter if needed. Once all the beef is browned, return it all to the pot. Stir in the tomato paste, garlic, bay leaf, and thyme, making sure to coat the beef. Cook for 1 minute, then slowly pour in 1 cup of the broth while scraping up the browned bits from the bottom of the pot. Add the remaining 3 cups broth and bring the stew to a simmer. Cover, reduce the heat to low, and simmer until the beef is tender (pierce with a fork to check), 10–15 minutes.

Add the onion, celery, carrots, tomatoes, and mushrooms and turn up the heat until it boils. Turn down the heat and simmer, uncovered, until the vegetables and meat are tender, 40 minutes to 1 hour. Discard the bay leaf. Season with the sea salt and black pepper and serve. Store leftovers in an airtight container in the fridge for up to 3 days.

SERVES 4
PREP TIME: 15 MINUTES
COOKING TIME: 2½ HOURS

CALORIES: 428
CARBS: 8
PROTEIN: 39
FAT: 27

SLOW COOKER CREAMY BRUSSELS SPROUTS

Brussels sprouts coated in a creamy sauce and topped with crispy bacon is what we're simmering in our slow cooker. We like to serve them up with whatever veggies and protein we have in our kitchen—good options include riced cauliflower, roasted sweet potato or butternut squash, and some grilled steak.

- 2 **tablespoons (30 g) butter, melted**
- ½ **cup (120 mL) chicken broth**
- 4 **cups (400 g) halved Brussels sprouts**
- 1 **medium (150 g) yellow onion, sliced**
- 3 **garlic cloves, minced**
- 1 **teaspoon (5 mg) minced ginger**
- 1 **cup (225 g) cream cheese**
- 1 **teaspoon (5 g) sea salt**
- ½ **teaspoon (1 g) black pepper**
- 4 **bacon strips**
- ½ **cup (50 g) grated Parmesan cheese, for garnish**

  Chopped fresh parsley, for garnish

INSTRUCTIONS:

Combine the melted butter, chicken broth, Brussels sprouts, onion, garlic, ginger, cream cheese, sea salt, and black pepper in a slow cooker and stir well.

Cover and cook on low for 4 hours or on high for 2 hours.

When the Brussels sprouts are almost done, cook the bacon in a skillet over medium heat until crispy, 5–7 minutes. Transfer the bacon to a plate. When cool enough to handle, crumble the bacon.

Serve the Brussels sprouts hot, topped with the crumbled bacon, Parmesan cheese, and parsley. Store leftovers in an airtight container in the fridge for up to 3 days.

SERVES 4
PREP TIME: 10 MINUTES
COOKING TIME: 2–4 HOURS

CALORIES: 359
CARBS: 16
PROTEIN: 15
FAT: 27

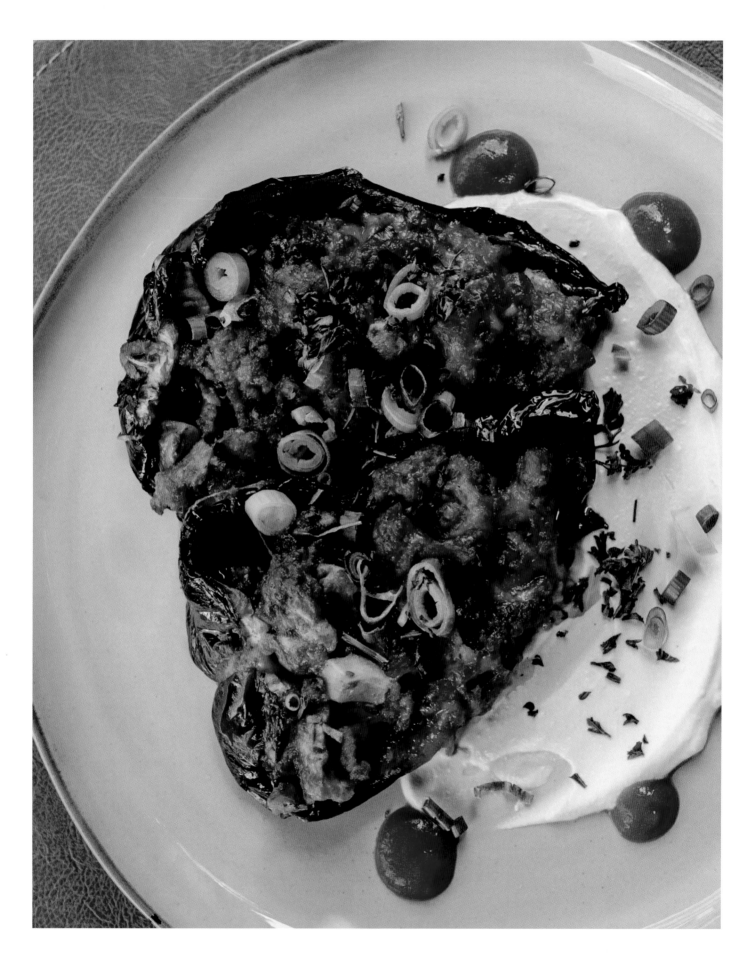

MEXICAN STUFFED POBLANO PEPPERS

These peppers are filled with a spicy pork and cheese mixture that everyone will love. Make these tonight and be sure to prepare enough to have leftovers!

- 1 pound (454) ground pork
- 2 teaspoons (10 g) sea salt
- 1 teaspoon (2 g) black pepper
- 1 teaspoon (5 g) smoked paprika
- 1 teaspoon (5 g) ground cumin
- ¼ cup (60 mL) extra-virgin olive oil, plus more for brushing
- 1 cup (114 g) shredded Mexican cheese, divided
- 1 medium (150 g) avocado, peeled, pitted, and diced
- 2 scallions, minced
- 4 large (70 g) poblano peppers, halved and seeded

GARNISH

- ¼ cup (60 g) full-fat sour cream
- Sliced scallions
- Minced fresh parsley
- Hot sauce

INSTRUCTIONS:

Preheat the broiler with a rack 4 inches from the heating element. Line a rimmed baking sheet with aluminum foil.

In a large skillet, cook the ground pork over medium heat, crumbling the meat, until no longer pink, 5–7 minutes. Drain off the fat. Season the meat with the sea salt, black pepper, smoked paprika, and cumin.

Stir in the olive oil, ½ cup of the shredded cheese, the diced avocado, and the scallions.

Place the peppers on the prepared baking sheet, cut sides down, and brush with olive oil. Broil the peppers until the skins blister, about 5 minutes.

Turn the peppers over with a pair of tongs. Fill with the ground pork mixture and sprinkle with the remaining ½ cup cheese. Broil until the cheese has melted, about 1–2 minutes longer. Garnish with sour cream, scallions, parsley, and dollops of hot sauce and serve.

SERVES 4	CALORIES: 505
PREP TIME: 10 MINUTES	CARBS: 10
COOKING TIME: 15 MINUTES	PROTEIN: 26
	FAT: 39

ROASTED DIJON SAUSAGE AND VEGGIES

This sheet pan recipe makes life easy. We love the Dijon vinaigrette these Italian sausage slices and veggies are coated in!

- ¼ cup (60 g) extra-virgin olive oil
- Grated zest of ½ lemon
- 1 tablespoon (15 mL) fresh lemon juice
- 1 tablespoon (15 g) Dijon mustard
- 1 teaspoon (5 g) sea salt
- ½ teaspoon (1 g) black pepper
- 1 tablespoon (15 g) Italian seasoning
- ½ teaspoon (2.5 g) red pepper flakes
- 1 pound (454 g) Italian sausage
- 1 medium (150 g) onion, chopped
- 3 garlic cloves, minced
- 2 medium (100 g) carrots, peeled and diced
- 2 cups (180 g) chopped Brussels sprouts
- 2 medium (228 g) sweet potatoes, diced
- Minced fresh parsley, for garnish
- ½ cup (50 g) grated Parmesan cheese, for garnish

INSTRUCTIONS:

Preheat the oven to 400°F (200°C). Line a rimmed baking sheet with parchment paper.

Whisk together the olive oil, lemon zest and juice, Dijon mustard, sea salt, black pepper, Italian seasoning, and red pepper flakes in a bowl or measuring cup with a spout. Set aside.

Arrange the Italian sausage on the prepared baking sheet. Scatter the onion, garlic, carrots, Brussels sprouts, and sweet potatoes around the sausage. Drizzle the olive oil mixture over everything.

Roast until the veggies are soft, the sausage is cooked through, and everything has begun to brown, about 30 minutes, tossing after 15 minutes.

Serve, garnished with fresh parsley and grated Parmesan cheese.

SERVES 4
PREP TIME: 15 MINUTES
COOKING TIME: 30 MINUTES

CALORIES: 670
CARBS: 24
PROTEIN: 24
FAT: 53

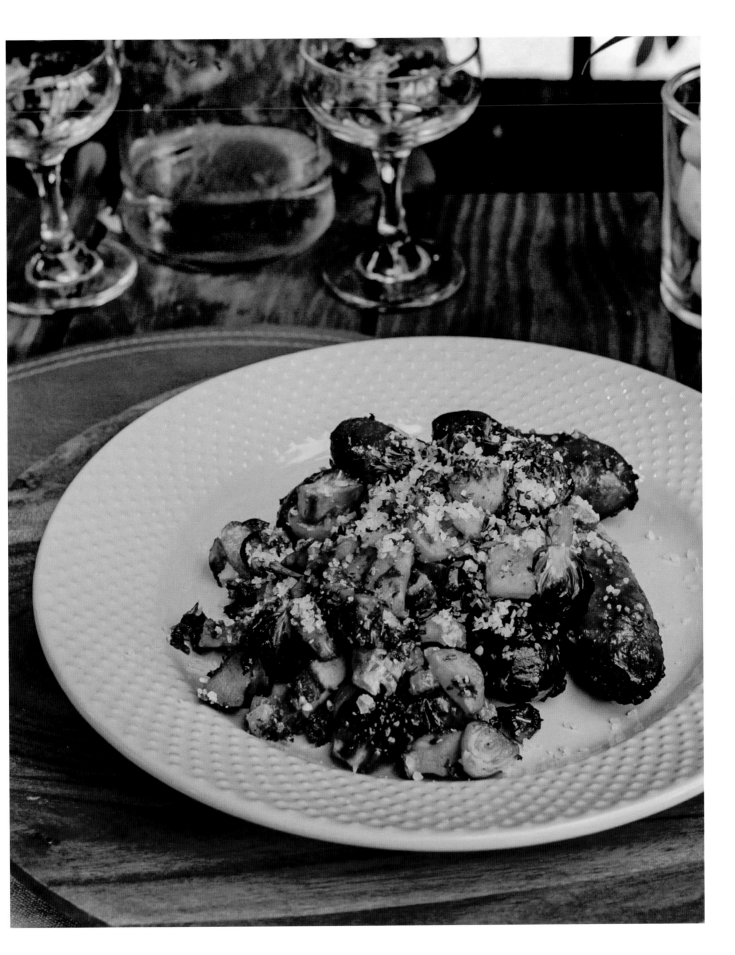

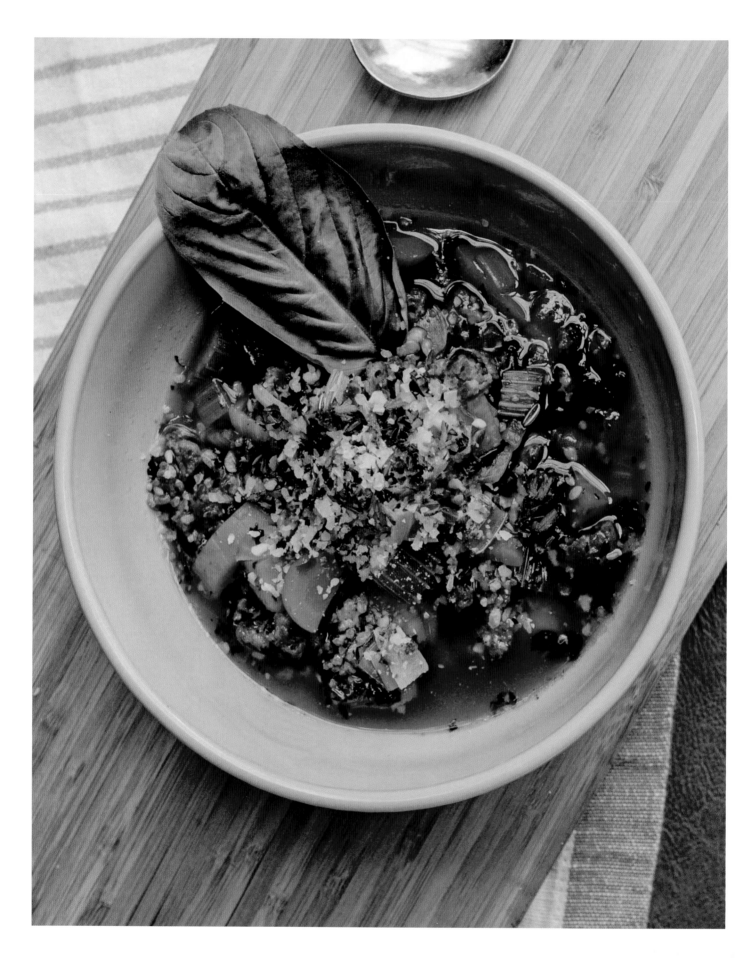

ITALIAN SAUSAGE AND SWEET POTATO SOUP

Make this big pot of soup to enjoy on a colder evening and get ready to be comforted! Throw in whatever leafy greens you have on hand to increase the veggies in this delicious one-pot meal.

- 2 tablespoons (30 g) butter
- 1 pound (454 g) Italian sausage, removed from casings and crumbled
- 1 medium (150 g) onion, minced
- 3 garlic cloves, minced
- 2 medium (100 g) celery stalks, diced
- 2 medium (100 g) carrots, peeled and cut into half-moons
- 4 cups (960 mL) chicken stock or bone broth
- 2 medium (228 g) sweet potatoes, peeled and diced
- 1 teaspoon (5 g) sea salt
- 1 tablespoon (15 g) Italian seasoning
- 1 bay leaf
- 1 teaspoon (5 g) fennel seeds
- ½ teaspoon (2.5 g) red pepper flakes
- Minced fresh parsley or basil, for garnish
- ½ cup (50 g) grated Parmesan cheese, for garnish

INSTRUCTIONS:

Melt the butter in a large stockpot over medium heat. Add the crumbled sausage and sauté, stirring and breaking up the meat, until lightly browned, 5–6 minutes. Use a slotted spoon to transfer the sausage to a plate.

Add the onion, garlic, celery, and carrots to the pan and stir to combine. Sauté for 5 minutes, stirring occasionally.

Add the chicken stock, sweet potatoes, sea salt, Italian seasoning, bay leaf, fennel seeds, red pepper flakes, and cooked sausage and stir well to combine. Bring the soup to a simmer, then reduce the heat to medium-low, cover, and simmer until the sweet potatoes are cooked through and tender, about 15 minutes.

Discard the bay leaf. Serve garnished with fresh parsley or basil and grated Parmesan cheese.

SERVES 4
PREP TIME: 15 MINUTES
COOKING TIME: 30 MINUTES

CALORIES: 656
CARBS: 23
PROTEIN: 32
FAT: 52

ITALIAN SAUSAGE STUFFED SWEET POTATOES

Sweet potatoes are such a treat, especially when stuffed with browned ground pork, sun-dried tomatoes, and tasty garnishes such as fresh herbs, walnuts, and Parmesan cheese. You can swap in any meat in this recipe, such as ground beef, chicken, or turkey; if you use a leaner meat, be sure to add a little healthier fat, such as first cold-press extra-virgin olive oil, to your garnishes.

- 4 **medium (454 g) sweet potatoes, well scrubbed**
- 5 **tablespoons (75 g) butter, divided**
- 1 **medium (150 g) onion, minced**
- 2 **garlic cloves, minced**
- 1 **pound (454 g) ground pork**
- 2 **teaspoons (10 g) sea salt, divided**
- ½ **teaspoon (1 g) black pepper**
- 1 **teaspoon (5 g) fennel seeds**
- ½ **teaspoon (2.5 g) red pepper flakes**
- ¼ **cup (60 g) sun-dried tomatoes, packed in olive oil, chopped**

GARNISH:

- **Minced fresh parsley or basil**
- ¼ **cup (28 g) chopped walnuts**
- ¼ **cup (25 g) grated Parmesan cheese**

INSTRUCTIONS:

Preheat the oven to 400°F (200°C).

Wrap each sweet potato in aluminum foil. Bake directly on an oven rack until very soft, 40–50 minutes.

While the sweet potatoes are baking, melt 1 tablespoon of the butter in a skillet over medium heat. Add the onion and garlic and sauté until soft, about 5 minutes. Add the ground pork and season with 1 teaspoon of the sea salt, the black pepper, fennel seeds, and red pepper flakes. Cook, stirring to break up the meat, until slightly brown, about 10 minutes. Turn off the heat and stir in the sun-dried tomatoes.

When the sweet potatoes are done, remove them from the oven and allow to cool a bit, then unwrap. Slit each potato down its center, place 1 tablespoon of the remaining butter in each potato and allow it to melt, then season all 4 potatoes with the remaining 1 teaspoon sea salt.

Stuff each sweet potato with the Italian sausage mixture and garnish with fresh parsley or basil, chopped walnuts, and grated Parmesan cheese.

SERVES 4		CALORIES: 637
PREP TIME: 15 MINUTES		CARBS: 27
COOKING TIME: 1 HOUR		PROTEIN: 26
		FAT: 46

CINNAMON BEEF AND GREENS

Cinnamon is an unexpected addition to ground beef, but it sure is delicious! This dish is warming and comforting without compromising your health goals, so dig in!

- 2 tablespoons (30 g) butter
- 1 pound (454 g) ground beef
- Grated zest of ½ lemon
- 1 teaspoon (5 g) sea salt
- ½ teaspoon (1 g) black pepper
- ½ teaspoon (0.7 g) garlic powder
- 1 teaspoon (5 g) red pepper flakes
- 1 teaspoon (5 g) fennel seeds
- 1 teaspoon (5 g) dried thyme
- 2 teaspoons (10 g) ground cinnamon
- Pinch ground cloves
- 1 (10-ounce/284 g) package frozen spinach
- 1 cup (240 mL) heavy cream
- Chopped fresh cilantro, for garnish

INSTRUCTIONS:

Melt the butter in a large skillet over medium-low heat. Add the ground beef and cook, stirring to break up the meat, until cooked through, about 10 minutes. Season with the lemon zest, sea salt, black pepper, garlic powder, red pepper flakes, fennel seeds, thyme, cinnamon, and cloves. Stir well to combine.

Add the frozen spinach to the skillet and stir to defrost and cook it, about 5 minutes. Stir in the cream, bring to a simmer, and cook until the entire mixture is thickened and creamy. Garnish with fresh cilantro and serve.

SERVES 4
PREP TIME: 5 MINUTES
COOKING TIME: 20 MINUTES

CALORIES: 553
CARBS: 8
PROTEIN: 23
FAT: 46

MEAT, CHEESE, AND VEGGIE BOWLS

This dish proves that eating keto can be simple and fast, as it is all cooked in one skillet and is done in just 15 minutes. Feel free to use cheeses other than pepper Jack—we just happen to like the bit of kick that it provides to this meal!

- 2 **tablespoons (30 g) butter**
- 1 **pound (454 g) ground pork**
- 2 **garlic cloves, minced**
- 1 **medium (124 g) zucchini, trimmed and cut into half-moons**
- 1 **cup (100 g) cremini mushrooms, sliced**
- 1 **teaspoon (5 g) sea salt**
- ½ **teaspoon (1 g) black pepper**
- 1 **tablespoon (15 g) fennel seeds**
- 1 **cup (149 g) cherry tomatoes, halved**
- 1 **cup (114 g) grated pepper Jack cheese**

INSTRUCTIONS:

Melt the butter in a skillet over medium heat. Add the ground pork and garlic and cook, stirring often to break up the meat, until browned, about 10 minutes. Using a slotted spoon, transfer the pork to a plate, reserving the grease in the skillet.

Add the zucchini and mushrooms to the skillet, season with the sea salt, black pepper, and fennel seeds, and sauté until the veggies are soft, about 5 minutes. Stir in the cherry tomatoes and the browned ground pork.

Turn off the heat, scatter the grated cheese over the top, and cover the skillet to allow the cheese to melt before serving.

SERVES 4
PREP TIME: **10 MINUTES**
COOKING TIME: **15 MINUTES**

CALORIES: **497**
CARBS: **8**
PROTEIN: **29**
FAT: **39**

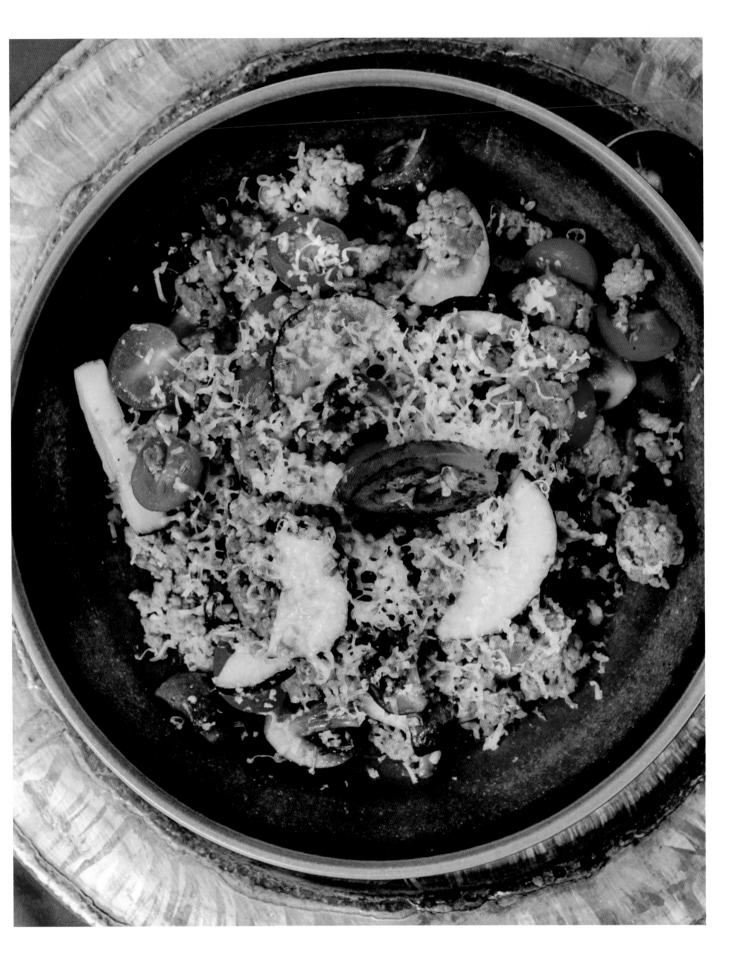

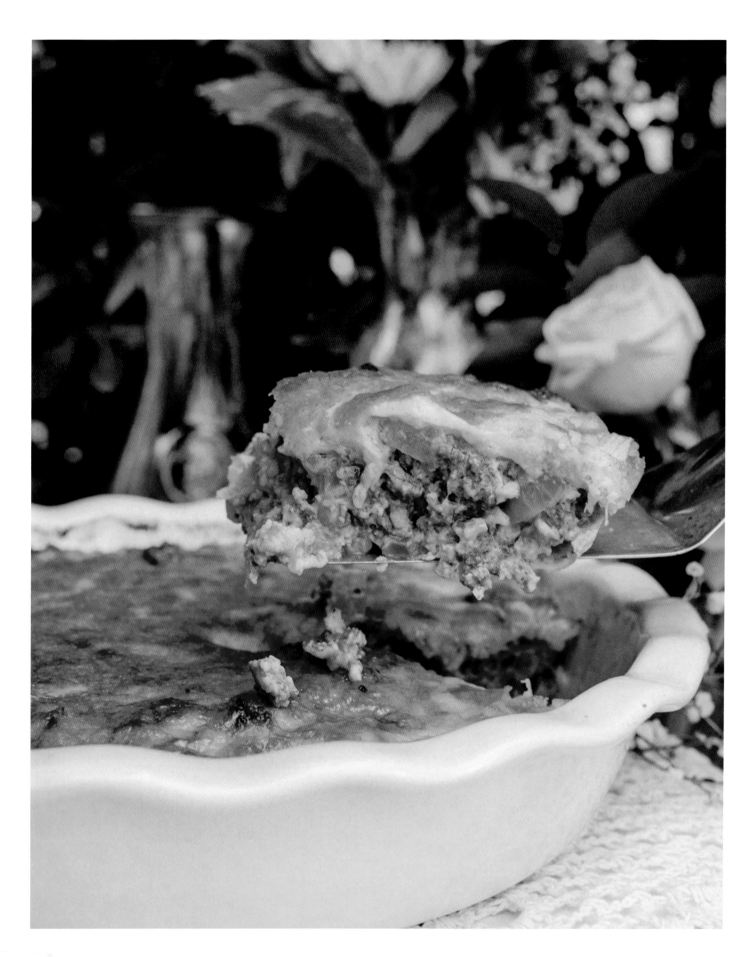

BACON CHEESEBURGER CASSEROLE

Make this extra-special casserole for a big group of loved ones and feel free to get fancy with added toppings such as diced tomato, diced avocado, minced scallion, or a sprinkle of smoked paprika!

8   bacon strips

1   **pound (454 g) ground beef**

1   **medium (150 g) yellow onion, minced**

3   **garlic cloves, minced**

4   **large eggs**

4   **ounces (114 g) heavy cream**

2   **teaspoons (10 g) sea salt**

1   **teaspoon (2 g) black pepper**

1   **teaspoon (5 g) red pepper flakes**

    Pinch ground nutmeg

2   **cups (228 g) shredded Cheddar cheese, divided**

INSTRUCTIONS:

Preheat the oven to 350°F (180°C).

Cook the bacon in a skillet over medium heat until crispy, 5–7 minutes. Transfer the bacon to a plate, leaving the grease in the skillet.

Add the ground beef, onion, and garlic to the same skillet and cook over medium-high heat until the meat is cooked through and crumbly, 5–7 minutes. Drain off the grease.

Spread the beef in the bottom of a 9 × 13-inch baking pan or similar. Crumble the bacon on top.

In a medium bowl, whisk together the eggs, cream, sea salt, black pepper, red pepper flakes, and nutmeg. Stir in 1 cup of the shredded cheese.

Pour the egg mixture over the beef and bacon. Top with the remaining 1 cup shredded cheese.

Bake until golden brown on top, 35–40 minutes.

SERVES 6
PREP TIME: 15 MINUTES
COOKING TIME: 50 MINUTES

CALORIES: 510
CARBS: 4
PROTEIN: 31
FAT: 41

GRILLED RIBEYE STEAKS WITH HERBED BUTTER

In this recipe we transform regular ol' butter (which is amazing as is!) into something truly extra special by mixing in fresh herbs, spices, and lemon zest. Then we serve it with a delicious grilled ribeye steak. So, who's coming over for dinner? We'll save you a seat.

HERBED BUTTER:

- ½ cup (1 stick/114 g) butter
- 1 scallion, minced
- ¼ cup (16 g) fresh parsley leaves
- ¼ cup (16 g) fresh cilantro leaves
- Grated zest of ½ lemon
- ½ teaspoon (1 g) black pepper
- 1 teaspoon (5 g) red pepper flakes

MARINADE:

- 2 garlic cloves, minced
- 1 teaspoon (5 g) sea salt
- ½ teaspoon (1 g) black pepper
- ½ teaspoon (5 g) ground ginger
- 1 teaspoon (5 g) red pepper flakes
- 1 tablespoon (15 mL) fresh lime juice
- 2 tablespoons (30 mL) coconut aminos

STEAKS:

- 1 pound (454 g) ribeye steaks
- Mixed greens, for serving

INSTRUCTIONS:

Combine all the herbed butter ingredients in a food processor and pulse until well combined. Scoop out the butter mixture and form into a log with your hands. Place on a plate and refrigerate while you prepare the steaks.

Combine all the marinade ingredients in a zip-top bag and add the steaks. Seal, making sure the steaks are well coated with the marinade. Let the meat marinate at room temperature for 15 minutes.

Heat the grill to medium heat. Remove the steaks from the marinade and grill to your desired doneness (for medium-rare, a thermometer should read 135°F; for medium, 140°F; for medium-well, 145°F).

Slice the chilled herbed butter into 1-inch slices. Slice the steak. Top with the herbed butter. Allow the butter to melt into the steaks and serve over the mixed greens.

SERVES 4
PREP TIME: 20 MINUTES
COOKING TIME: 15 MINUTES

CALORIES: 464
CARBS: 4
PROTEIN: 23
FAT: 30

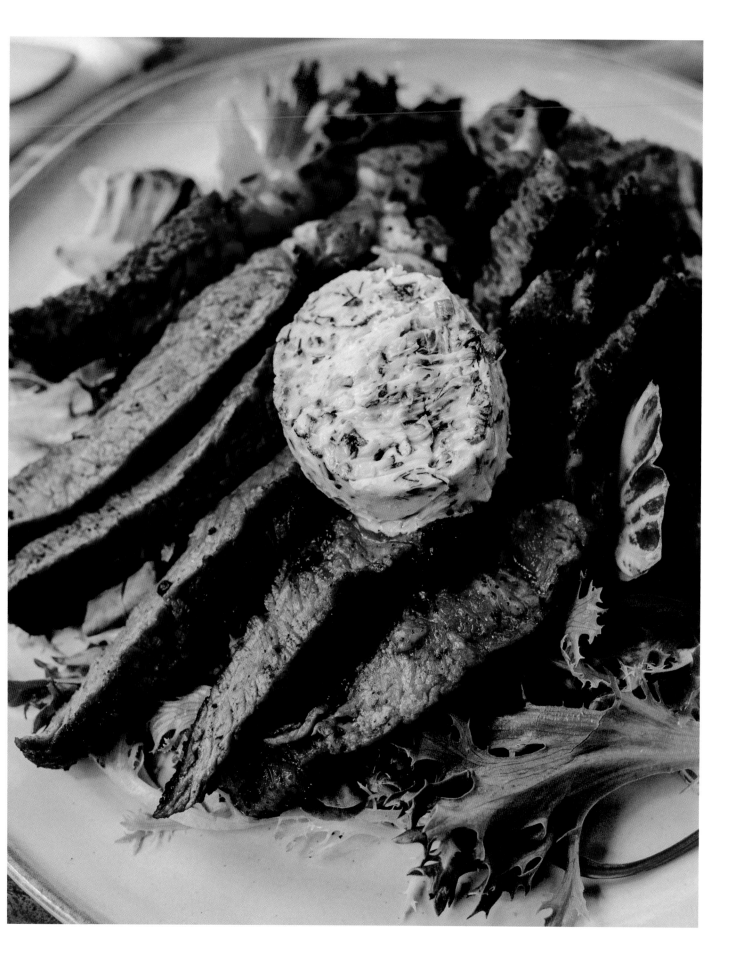

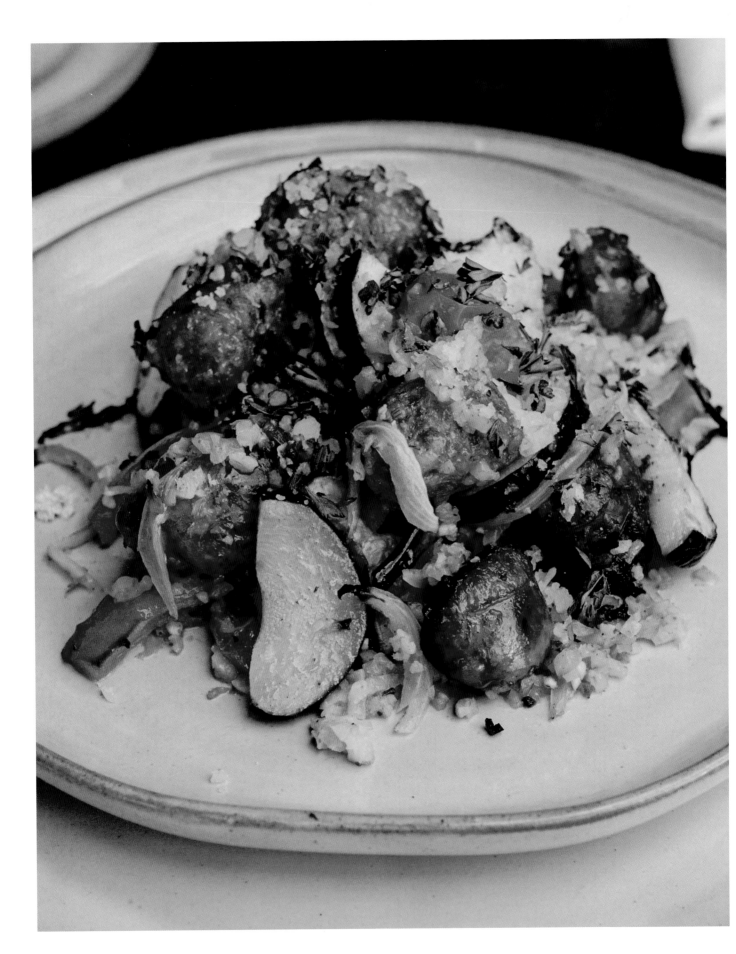

SMOKED SAUSAGE AND VEGGIE BAKE

This dish is a cinch to prepare—just arrange everything on a big baking sheet and stick it in the oven until browned. It's sure to become a family favorite!

- 4 (5-ounce/143 g) smoked sausages, cut into ½-inch slices
- 1 medium (150 g) yellow onion, sliced
- 1 cup (150 g) cherry tomatoes
- 1 medium (150 g) red bell pepper, seeded and sliced
- 1 medium (190 g) zucchini, trimmed and sliced
- 2 cups (500 g) riced cauliflower
- 2 garlic cloves, minced

- ¼ cup (60 mL) extra-virgin olive oil
- 2 teaspoons (10 g) sea salt
- 1 teaspoon (2 g) black pepper
- 1 teaspoon (5 g) smoked paprika

OPTIONAL:

- Minced fresh parsley, for garnish
- 1 medium (150 g) avocado, peeled, pitted, and diced, for garnish

INSTRUCTIONS:

Preheat the oven to 400°F (200°C). Line a rimmed baking sheet with parchment paper.

Combine the sausages and all the vegetables on the prepared baking sheet. Drizzle the olive oil over everything, season with the sea salt, black pepper, and smoked paprika, and toss well to combine. Spread everything out in a single layer.

Bake until the sausage is cooked through and the veggies are soft and have begun to brown, 25–30 minutes. Serve with minced parsley and avocado (optional).

SERVES 4
PREP TIME: 10 MINUTES
COOKING TIME: 30 MINUTES

CALORIES: 298
CARBS: 11
PROTEIN: 6
FAT: 25

SLOW-COOKED BEEF TACO SOUP

Just add these ingredients to a slow cooker and in a few hours you will have a delicious, creamy soup with all of the taco flavors you love! Mixing in cream cheese when this is done makes this extra special and comforting.

- 1 **pound (454 g) ground beef**
- 1 **medium (150 g) yellow onion, diced**
- 4 **garlic cloves, minced**
- 1 **jalapeño, seeded and minced**
- 2 **teaspoons (10 g) sea salt**
- 1 **teaspoon (2 g) black pepper**
- 1 **tablespoon (15 g) ground cumin**
- 1 **teaspoon (5 g) chili powder**
- 1 **teaspoon (5 g) red pepper flakes**
- 2 **tablespoons (30 mL) fresh lime juice**
- 2 **cups (480 mL) beef stock**
- 1 **cup (240 g) canned diced fire-roasted tomatoes**
- 8 **ounces (228 g) cream cheese**

Minced fresh cilantro, for garnish

- ½ **cup (56 g) shredded Cheddar cheese, for garnish**

INSTRUCTIONS:

Crumble the ground beef into the slow cooker and add the onion, garlic, jalapeño, sea salt, black pepper, cumin, chili powder, red pepper flakes, lime juice, beef stock, and diced tomatoes with their juices. Cover and cook on low for 4 hours.

Add the cream cheese and whisk constantly until the cream cheese is fully melted and incorporated. Garnish with fresh cilantro and shredded cheese and serve.

SERVES 4
PREP TIME: 10 MINUTES
COOKING TIME: 4 HOURS

CALORIES: 585
CARBS: 12
PROTEIN: 31
FAT: 46

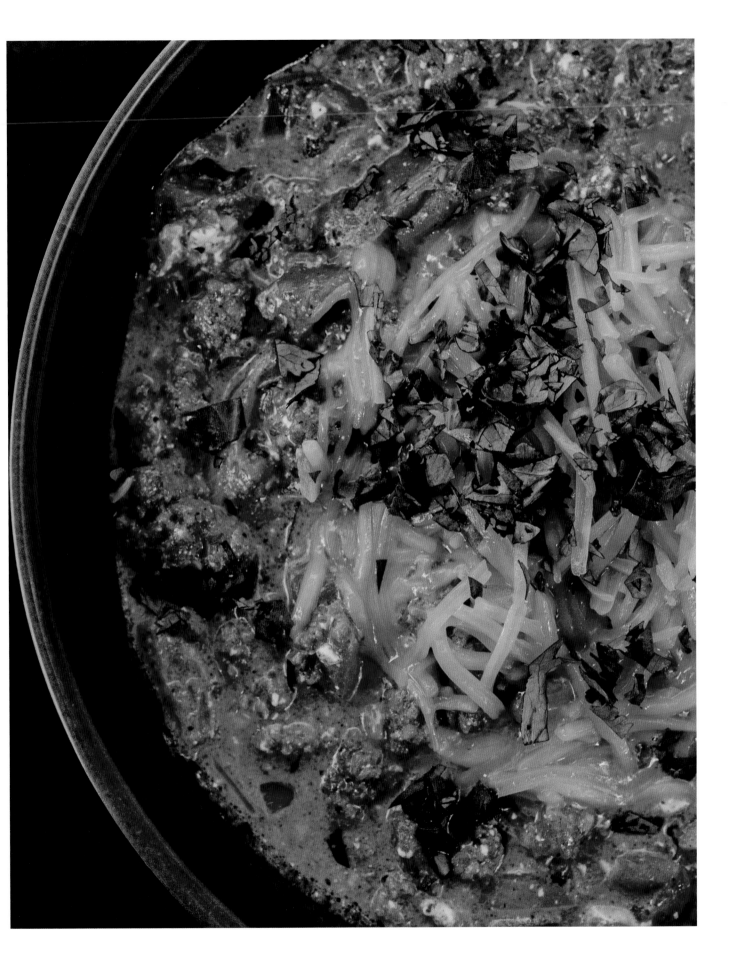

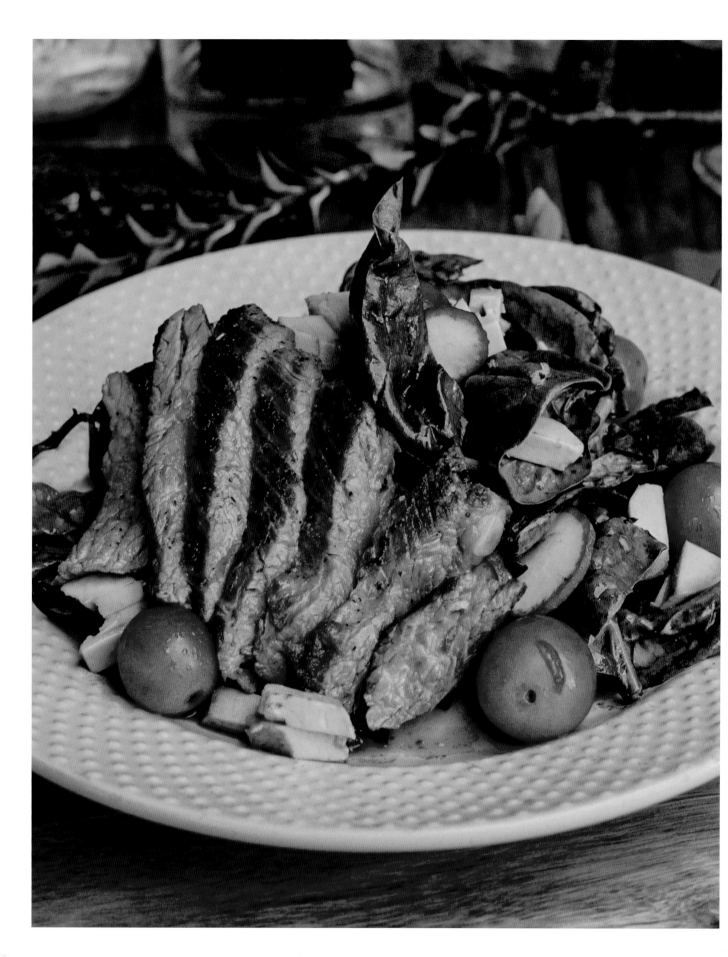

FLAT-IRON STEAK SALAD

This steak salad takes just minutes to prepare but will leave you feeling satisfied between meals so you can accomplish all the things you've been daydreaming about—you know what they are!

STEAK:

- 12 ounces (342 g) flat-iron steak
- ½ teaspoon (2.5 g) sea salt
- ¼ teaspoon (0.5 g) black pepper

VINAIGRETTE:

- ¼ cup (60 mL) extra-virgin olive oil
- 2 tablespoons (30 mL) balsamic vinegar
- 1 tablespoon (15 mL) fresh lemon juice
- 1 teaspoon (5 g) sea salt
- ½ teaspoon (1 g) black pepper

SALAD:

- 6 cups (180 g) baby spinach
- 16 cherry tomatoes
- 1 medium (150 g) avocado, peeled, pitted, and diced
- 4 radishes, sliced

OPTIONAL:

- ½ cup (230 g) crumbled blue cheese

INSTRUCTIONS:

Heat the grill to medium heat. Sprinkle the steak with the sea salt and black pepper. Grill the steak to your desired doneness (for medium-rare, a thermometer should read 135°F; for medium, 140°F; for medium-well, 145°F). Let stand for 5 minutes.

In a small bowl, whisk together all the vinaigrette ingredients.

Divide the spinach among 4 plates. Add the tomatoes, avocado, and radishes.

Slice the steak and place over the salad. Drizzle with the vinaigrette. Optional: Sprinkle the blue cheese on top.

SERVES 4	CALORIES: 334
PREP TIME: 10 MINUTES	CARBS: 7
COOKING TIME: 15 MINUTES	PROTEIN: 20
	FAT: 25

ROSEMARY-GARLIC PORK CHOPS

Infusing butter with garlic and fresh rosemary and smothering it on top of pork chops and a batch of riced cauliflower will leave you feeling fit as a fiddle so you can focus on your goals with much more ease.

4   (4-ounce/114 g) pork loin chops

2   teaspoons (10 g) sea salt

1   teaspoon (2 g) black pepper

½   cup (1 stick/114 g) butter, melted

2   garlic cloves, minced

1   tablespoon (15 g) minced fresh rosemary

2   tablespoons (30 mL) extra-virgin olive oil

1   pound (454 g) riced cauliflower

INSTRUCTIONS:

Preheat the oven to 375°F (190°C).

Sprinkle the pork chops with the sea salt and black pepper.

In a small bowl mix together the melted butter, garlic, and rosemary. Set aside.

Heat the olive oil in a cast-iron skillet over medium-high heat, then add the pork chops. Sear until golden, about 4 minutes, then flip and cook for 4 minutes more. Brush the pork chops generously with the garlic butter, reserving the remainder for serving.

Add the riced cauliflower and stir around the pork chops, allowing the garlic butter to coat the riced cauliflower.

Place the skillet in the oven and bake until the pork chops are cooked through (145°F/65°C for medium), 10–12 minutes. Serve with the remaining garlic butter.

SERVES 4
PREP TIME: 10 MINUTES
COOKING TIME: 20 MINUTES

CALORIES: 503
CARBS: 4
PROTEIN: 24
FAT: 44

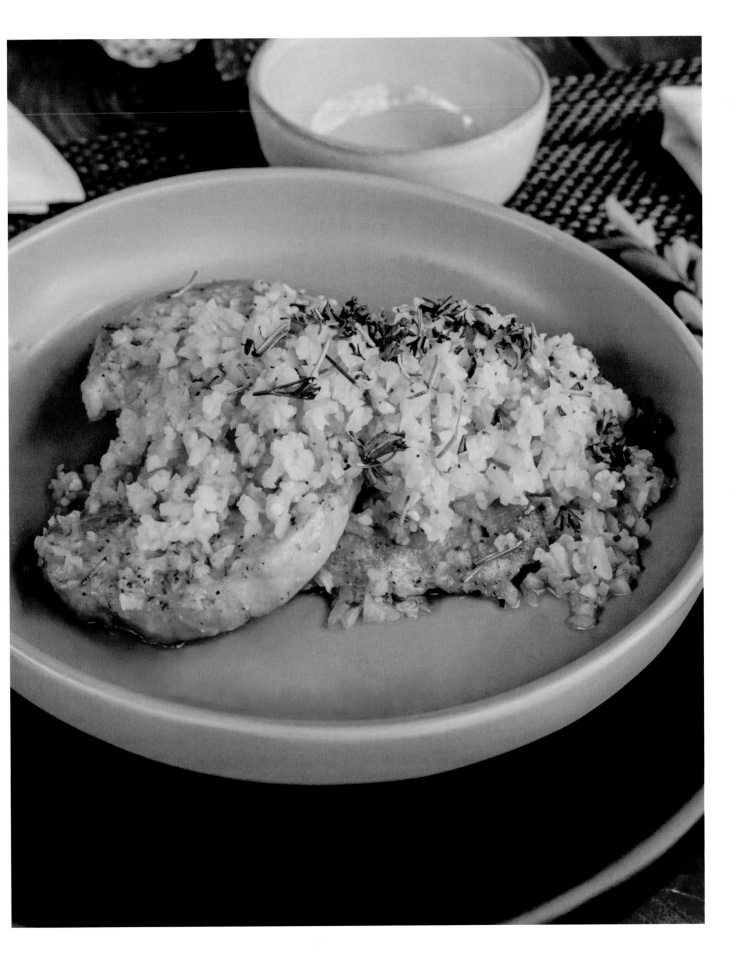

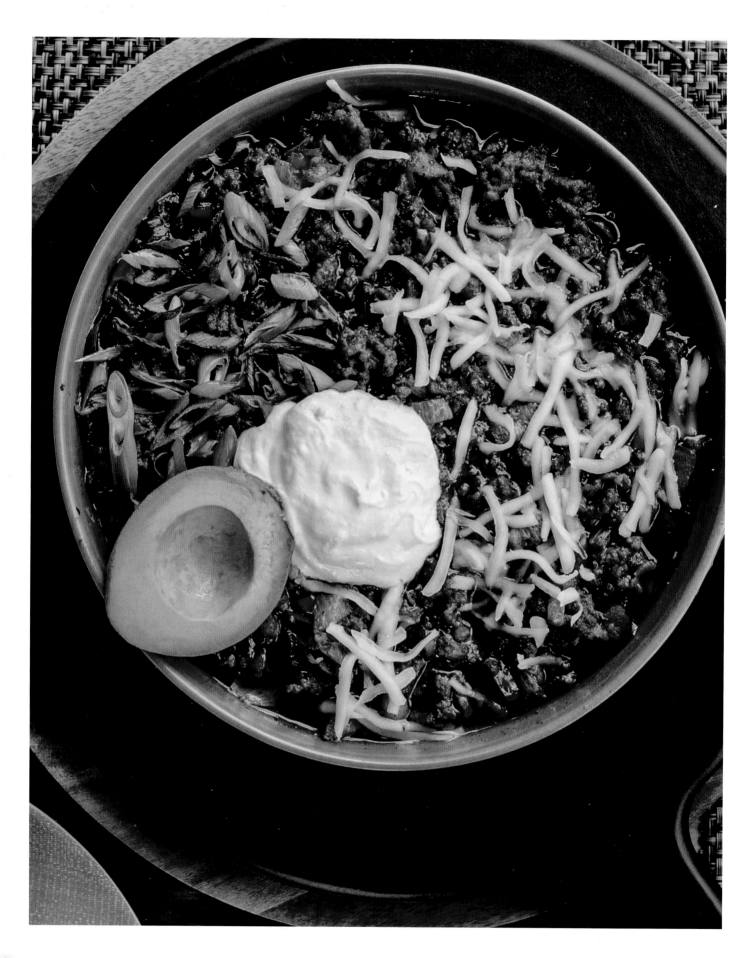

BEEF CHILI

A big batch of beef chili will hit the spot after a day of activity and knocking out items on your to-do list. You can stick portions of this in the freezer so that you can quickly grab and reheat for those days that are extra packed!

- 4 bacon strips
- 1 medium (150 g) yellow onion, diced
- 2 medium (100 g) celery stalks, diced
- 1 medium (150 g) red bell pepper, seeded and diced
- ½ cup (50 g) cremini mushrooms, chopped
- 2 garlic cloves, minced
- 1 pound (454 g) ground beef
- 2 tablespoons (30 g) chili powder
- 1 tablespoon (15 g) ground cumin
- 1 tablespoon (15 g) dried oregano
- 1 tablespoon (15 g) smoked paprika
- 2 teaspoons (10 g) sea salt
- 1 teaspoon (2 g) black pepper

- 2 cups (480 mL) beef stock
- ¼ cup (60 g) full-fat sour cream
- ¼ cup (28 g) shredded cheese
- Sliced scallion
- 2 medium (300 g) avocados, peeled, pitted, and halved

INSTRUCTIONS:

Cook the bacon in a large pot over medium heat until crispy, 5–7 minutes. Transfer the bacon to a plate, leaving the grease in the pot. When cool enough to handle, crumble the bacon and stir it back into the dish after the liquid has evaporated.

Add the onion, celery, bell pepper, and mushrooms to the pot and cook until soft, about 6 minutes. Add the garlic and cook until fragrant, about 1 minute more.

Push the vegetables to one side of the pot and add the beef. Cook, stirring occasionally to break up the meat, until no pink remains, 5–7 minutes.

Add the chili powder, cumin, oregano, paprika, sea salt, and black pepper. Stir to combine and cook for 2 minutes more. Add the beef stock and bring to a simmer. Cook until most of the liquid has evaporated, 10–15 minutes.

Serve in bowls and top with the sour cream, shredded cheese, sliced scallion, and halved avocado.

SERVES 4
PREP TIME: 10 MINUTES
COOKING TIME: 30 MINUTES

CALORIES: 497
CARBS: 11
PROTEIN: 32
FAT: 36

CHEESY BUTTERNUT SQUASH BAKE

This comforting dish is festive enough to make for a holiday, but we often make it on regular weeknights and no one is complaining! To bulk this up, add a big handful of baby spinach and sautéed mushrooms.

- 4 **bacon strips**
- 1 **pound (454 g) ground pork**
- 4 **cups (500 g) peeled and cubed butternut squash**
- 2 **garlic cloves, minced**
- 2 **teaspoons (10 g) sea salt**
- 1 **teaspoon (2 g) black pepper**
- 1 **teaspoon (5 g) fennel seeds**
- 1 **teaspoon (5 g) red pepper flakes**
- 1 **teaspoon (5 g) dried thyme**
- 1 **cup (100 g) grated Parmesan cheese**
- ½ **cup (56 g) shredded mozzarella cheese**
- **Minced fresh parsley, for garnish**

INSTRUCTIONS:

Preheat the oven to 425°F (220°C).

Cook the bacon in a large skillet over medium heat until crispy, 5–7 minutes. Transfer the bacon to a plate, leaving the grease in the skillet. When cool enough to handle, crumble the bacon.

Add the ground pork to the same skillet, and cook, stirring to break up the meat, until no longer pink, 5–7 minutes. Add the butternut squash and garlic and season with the sea salt, black pepper, fennel seeds, red pepper flakes, and thyme. Transfer the skillet to the oven and bake until the squash is tender, 20–25 minutes.

Remove the skillet from the oven and top with the Parmesan and mozzarella. Bake until the cheese is melty, another 5–10 minutes. Garnish with the crumbled bacon and minced parsley and serve.

SERVES 4
PREP TIME: **10 MINUTES**
COOKING TIME: **35 MINUTES**

CALORIES: **604**
CARBS: **20**
PROTEIN: **28**
FAT: **47**

ZUCCHINI JALAPEÑO BAKE

Jalapeño gives this dish some heat, so use less if you prefer a milder flavor—or more if you like things extra hot! Using ground pork instead of leaner cuts ensures more healthy fats in your diet, not to mention how delicious it is.

- 4 **bacon strips**
- 1 **pound (454 g) ground pork**
- 4 **medium (500 g) zucchini, trimmed and diced**
- 2 **garlic cloves, minced**
- 2 **teaspoons (10 g) sea salt**
- 1 **teaspoon (2 g) black pepper**
- 1 **teaspoon (5 g) fennel seeds**
- 1 **teaspoon (5 g) red pepper flakes**
- 6 **ounces (170 g) cream cheese**
- 1 **jalapeño, seeded and minced**
- ½ **cup (56 g) shredded mozzarella cheese**
- ½ **cup (56 g) shredded Cheddar cheese**

Minced fresh parsley, for garnish

INSTRUCTIONS:

Preheat the oven to 425°F (220°C).

Cook the bacon in a large skillet over medium heat until crispy, 5–7 minutes. Transfer the bacon to a plate, leaving the grease in the skillet. When cool enough to handle, crumble the bacon.

Add the ground pork to the same skillet and cook, stirring to break up the meat, until no longer pink, 5–7 minutes. Add the zucchini and garlic and season with the sea salt, black pepper, fennel seeds, and red pepper flakes. Stir to combine everything.

Transfer the skillet to the oven and bake until the zucchini is tender, about 15 minutes. Remove the skillet from the oven, stir in the cream cheese and jalapeño, and top with the mozzarella and Cheddar. Bake until the cheese is melty, another 5–10 minutes.

Garnish with the crumbled bacon and minced parsley and serve.

SERVES 4
PREP TIME: 10 MINUTES
COOKING TIME: 35 MINUTES

CALORIES: 672
CARBS: 10
PROTEIN: 34
FAT: 55

PHILLY CHEESESTEAK BAKE

Whip this up when you want to enjoy the traditional flavors of a Philly cheesesteak sammie but don't want to compromise feeling strong and healthy. Fresh veggies, sirloin steak, and creamy cheese will hit the spot, no bread needed!

- 4 **tablespoons (60 mL) extra-virgin olive oil, divided**
- 1 **medium (150 g) yellow onion, sliced**
- 2 **garlic cloves, minced**
- 2 **medium (150 g) bell peppers (green and red), seeded and sliced**
- 1 **cup (100 g) sliced cremini mushrooms**
- 2 **teaspoons (10 g) sea salt, divided**
- 1 **teaspoon (2 g) black pepper, divided**
- 1 **pound (454 g) sirloin steak**
- ½ **cup (56 g) shredded mozzarella cheese**
- ½ **cup (56 g) shredded provolone cheese**
- **Minced fresh parsley, for garnish**

INSTRUCTIONS:

Preheat the oven to 350°F (180°C).

Heat 1 tablespoon of the olive oil in a large skillet over medium heat. Add the onion, garlic, bell peppers, and mushrooms and season with 1 teaspoon of the sea salt and ½ teaspoon of the black pepper. Cook, stirring often, until the vegetables are tender, about 5 minutes. Transfer the vegetables to a plate.

Add the remaining 3 tablespoons olive oil to the skillet and increase the heat to medium-high. Season the steak all over with the remaining 1 teaspoon sea salt and remaining ½ teaspoon black pepper and sear the steak, about 3 minutes per side. Turn off the heat and return the vegetables to the skillet.

Top everything with the mozzarella and provolone cheese. Bake until the peppers are tender and the cheese is melted, about 20 minutes. Garnish with minced parsley and serve.

SERVES 4
PREP TIME: 10 MINUTES
COOKING TIME: 35 MINUTES

CALORIES: 464
CARBS: 7
PROTEIN: 32
FAT: 34

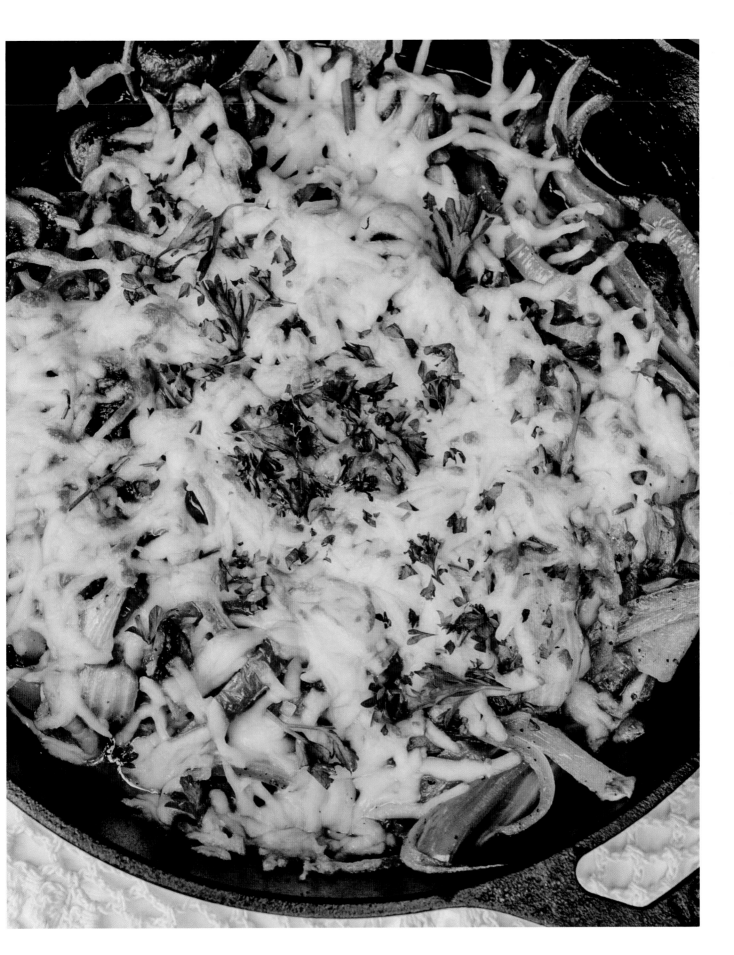

ZOODLES IN ALFREDO SAUCE

Get ready to impress with this recipe! Creamy and salty, this dish will hit the spot while leaving you feeling strong and healthy. Make a big batch to share with loved ones or to have as leftovers throughout the week.

4   **bacon strips**

½   **medium (75 g) yellow onion, minced**

2   **garlic cloves, minced**

¼   **cup (120 mL) dry white wine**

2   **cups (480 mL) heavy cream**

1   **cup (100 g) grated Parmesan cheese**

4   **cups (500 g) zucchini noodles**

2   **teaspoons (10 g) sea salt**

1   **teaspoon (2 g) freshly ground black pepper**

Minced fresh parsley, for garnish

INSTRUCTIONS:

Cook the bacon in a large skillet over medium heat until crispy, 5–7 minutes. Transfer the bacon to a plate, leaving the grease in the skillet. When cool enough to handle, crumble the bacon.

Add the onion to the skillet and cook until soft, about 2 minutes. Add the garlic and cook until fragrant, about 30 seconds. Add the wine and cook until reduced by half. Add the cream and bring the mixture to a boil. Reduce the heat to low and stir in the Parmesan cheese. Cook until the sauce has thickened slightly, about 2 minutes.

Add the zucchini noodles and toss until completely coated in the sauce. Remove from the heat and stir in the crumbled bacon. Season with the sea salt and black pepper, garnish with parsley, and serve.

SERVES 4	CALORIES: 667
PREP TIME: 10 MINUTES	CARBS: 13
COOKING TIME: 15 MINUTES	PROTEIN: 13
	FAT: 60

SLOW COOKER ZUPPA TOSCANA

No need for takeout when you can make your own Tuscan soup! Our version is low-carb and will leave you feeling satisfied and grounded in your body. If you don't have a slow cooker, simply simmer this soup in a Dutch oven over low heat for about an hour.

- 8 **ounces (228 g) mild or hot Italian sausage, removed from casings and crumbled**

- 1 **medium (150 g) yellow onion, diced**

- 2 **garlic cloves, minced**

- 2 **cups (480 mL) chicken stock**

- 4 **cups (400 g) cauliflower florets**

- 2 **cups (85 g) kale, chopped**

- 2 **teaspoons (10 g) sea salt**

- 1 **teaspoon (2 g) freshly ground black pepper**

- 1 **teaspoon (5 g) red pepper flakes**

- ½ **cup (120 mL) heavy cream**

  Minced fresh parsley, for garnish

INSTRUCTIONS:

Cook the ground sausage, onion, and garlic in a skillet over medium heat until cooked through, stirring often, 5–7 minutes. Transfer the sausage mixture (including the grease) to a slow cooker.

Add the chicken stock and cauliflower, kale, sea salt, black pepper, and red pepper flakes and mix until combined.

Cover and cook on high for 4 hours or on low for 6 hours.

Add the cream and mix until combined. Garnish with parsley and serve.

SERVES 2
PREP TIME: **10 MINUTES**
COOKING TIME: **4–6 HOURS**

CALORIES: **585**
CARBS: **21**
PROTEIN: **33**
FAT: **45**

BACON AND BLUE CHEESE STUFFED SQUASH

Spaghetti squash is made ultra-delicious by adding bacon, veggies, and cheese, making this meal a favorite for many. Eating forkfuls straight out of the squash shell will be a special memory for all those enjoying this dish together, so get this recipe on your menu soon!

- 1 **small spaghetti squash**
- 2 **tablespoons (30 mL) extra-virgin olive oil**
- 1 **teaspoon (5 g) sea salt**
- ½ **teaspoon (1 g) black pepper**
- 4 **bacon strips**
- 1 **cup (100 g) sliced cremini mushrooms**
- 2 **garlic cloves, minced**
- 2 **cups (60 g) baby spinach**
- ½ **cup (120 g) full-fat sour cream**
- ¼ **cup (115 g) crumbled blue cheese**

INSTRUCTIONS:

Preheat the oven to 400°F (200°C). Line a rimmed baking sheet with parchment paper.

Cut the squash in half lengthwise and scrape out the seeds. Brush the inside with the olive oil and sprinkle with the sea salt and black pepper.

Place the squash halves on the prepared baking sheet, cut side up, and bake until soft, about 45 minutes. Scrape the cooked flesh into a bowl and set aside. Return the spaghetti squash shells to the baking sheet.

While the squash is baking, cook the bacon in a skillet over medium heat until crispy, 5–7 minutes. Transfer the bacon to a plate, leaving the grease in the skillet. When cool enough to handle, crumble the bacon.

Add the mushrooms and garlic to the skillet and cook until soft, 4–5 minutes. Add the crumbled bacon and baby spinach. Stir until the spinach is wilted, about 2 minutes. Add the mushroom mixture to the bowl of squash. Mix in the sour cream and stir until the filling is combined.

Spoon the filling into the empty squash shells. Sprinkle each half with 2 tablespoons of the crumbled blue cheese. Bake until the cheese is melted and the squash is heated through, 4–5 minutes.

SERVES 2
PREP TIME: 5 MINUTES
COOKING TIME: 1 HOUR

CALORIES: 633
CARBS: 26
PROTEIN: 27
FAT: 51

BEEF EGG ROLL SLAW

This dish takes all the flavors of a traditional egg roll without the fluff, if you know what we mean! Cook this up to enjoy when you are craving some heat with your healthy fats and proteins that you've been feeding your body since going keto!

- 2 tablespoons (30 mL) toasted sesame oil
- ½ medium (150 g) yellow onion, diced
- 2 garlic cloves, minced
- 1 pound (454 g) ground beef
- 1 tablespoon (15 mL) sriracha
- 1 teaspoon (5 g) minced fresh ginger
- 1 teaspoon (5 g) sea salt
- ½ teaspoon (1 g) black pepper
- 4 cups (180 g) coleslaw mix or shredded cabbage
- 2 tablespoons (30 mL) coconut aminos
- 1 tablespoon (15 mL) raw apple cider vinegar
- 2 large eggs

GARNISH:

- 1 medium (150 g) avocado, peeled, pitted, and diced
- 1 scallion, minced
- Chopped fresh cilantro

INSTRUCTIONS:

Heat the sesame oil in a large skillet over medium-high heat. Add the onion and garlic and sauté until the onion is translucent and the garlic is fragrant, about 5 minutes. Add the ground beef, sriracha, ginger, sea salt, and black pepper and sauté, stirring to break up the meat, until the beef is browned, about 5 minutes. Stir in the coleslaw mix, coconut aminos, and cider vinegar. Sauté until the coleslaw is tender, about 4 minutes more.

Crack the eggs into the skillet and break up quickly, scrambling them with the entire dish until cooked through. Serve topped with the avocado, scallion, and cilantro.

SERVES 4
PREP TIME: 5 MINUTES
COOKING TIME: 20 MINUTES

CALORIES: 498
CARBS: 11
PROTEIN: 26
FAT: 37

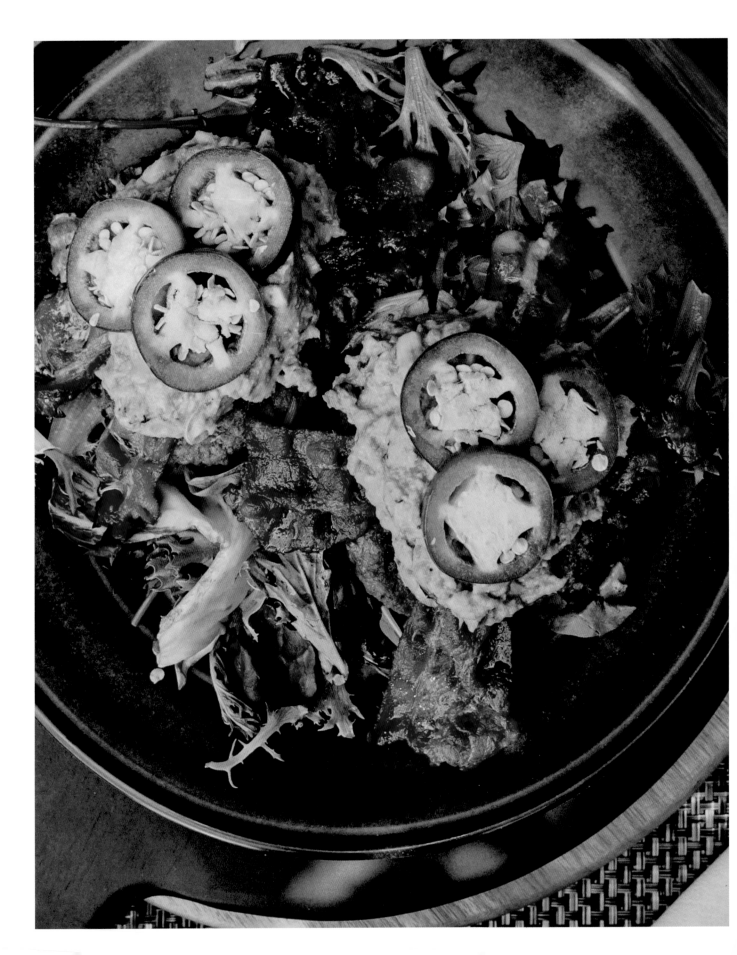

BACON GUACAMOLE BURGERS

What is better than burgers with bacon and guacamole? We can't think of anything, but let us know if you do, okay? Use any cheese in this recipe that you like. We opted for extra-sharp Cheddar, but any would be delicious—think feta, Swiss, or pepper Jack.

GUACAMOLE:

- 1 **medium (150 g) avocado, peeled, pitted, and diced**
- 1 **tablespoon (15 mL) fresh lime juice**
- ½ **teaspoon (2.5 g) sea salt**
- ¼ **teaspoon (0.3 g) garlic powder**
- **Chopped fresh cilantro to taste**

BURGERS:

- 8 **ounces (228 g) ground beef**
- 2 **garlic cloves, minced**
- 1 **teaspoon (5 g) sea salt**
- ½ **teaspoon (1 g) black pepper**
- ½ **teaspoon (2.5 g) onion powder**
- 4 **bacon strips**
- 2 **ounces (56 g) extra-sharp Cheddar cheese**
- 1 **jalapeño, seeded and sliced**
- 4 **cups (114 g) mixed greens**

INSTRUCTIONS:

Combine all the guacamole ingredients in a small bowl and mash with a fork until it is as smooth or as chunky as you like it. Set aside.

Gently mix the ground beef, garlic, sea salt, black pepper, and onion powder with your hands and form 2 patties. Set on a plate until ready to cook.

Cook the bacon in a cast-iron skillet over medium heat until crispy, 5–7 minutes. Transfer the bacon to a plate, leaving the grease in the skillet.

Place the burger patties in the skillet and cook until done to your liking, 4–5 minutes per side. Add the cheese slices to each patty, and turn off the heat. Place a lid on the skillet and allow the cheese to melt. Top the burgers with the bacon, guacamole, and jalapeño slices and serve on a bed of mixed greens.

SERVES **2**
PREP TIME: **10 MINUTES**
COOKING TIME: **15 MINUTES**

CALORIES: **528**
CARBS: **4**
PROTEIN: **33**
FAT: **41**

STEAK STIR-FRY WITH SNAP PEAS

A simple change of cooking fats, such as toasted sesame seed oil instead of olive oil, really transforms this dish, so be sure to keep a bottle in your pantry. Make this recipe just as noted below, or add some minced ginger and toasted cashews for a little something extra!

STIR-FRY:

- 2 tablespoons (30 mL) toasted sesame oil
- 2 tablespoons (30 mL) coconut aminos
- 1 tablespoon (15 mL) rice vinegar
- 2 garlic cloves, minced
- 1 teaspoon (5 g) sea salt
- ½ teaspoon (1 g) black pepper
- ½ teaspoon (2.5 g) onion powder
- 6 ounces (170 g) flank steak
- 1 medium (150 g) red bell pepper, seeded and sliced
- 1 cup (67 g) snap peas

GARNISH:

- 1 medium (150 g) avocado, peeled, pitted, and diced
- 2 teaspoons (10 mL) sriracha
- 2 teaspoons (10 g) sesame seeds
- Chopped fresh cilantro
- Fresh lime wedges

INSTRUCTIONS:

Combine the sesame oil, coconut aminos, rice vinegar, garlic, sea salt, black pepper, and onion powder in a shallow dish and whisk to combine. Cook the steak to medium-rare or medium as perferred, transfer it to a cutting board, and slice when cool enough to touch. Add the steak, bell pepper, and snap peas to the sesame oil mixture and let them marinate for 15 minutes.

Heat a cast-iron skillet over medium-high heat. When hot, add the steak and veggies with their marinade. Stir-fry until the veggies are soft and the steak is cooked through, 8–10 minutes. Top with the avocado, sriracha, sesame seeds, and cilantro and serve with lime wedges for squeezing.

SERVES 2
PREP TIME: 20 MINUTES
COOKING TIME: 10 MINUTES

CALORIES: 462
CARBS: 17
PROTEIN: 22
FAT: 32

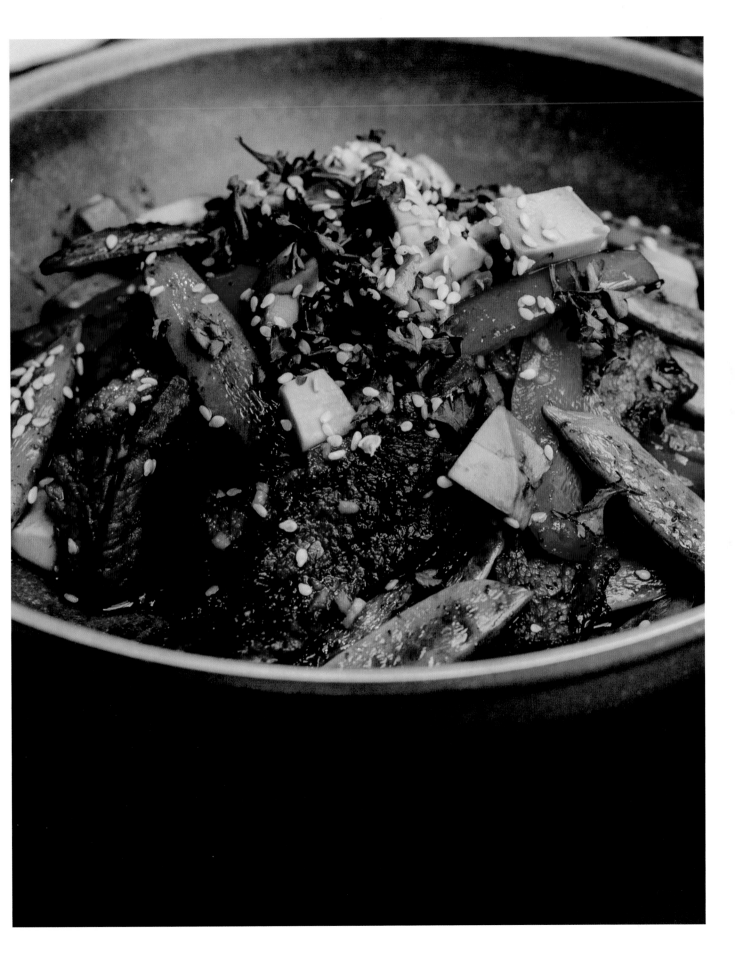

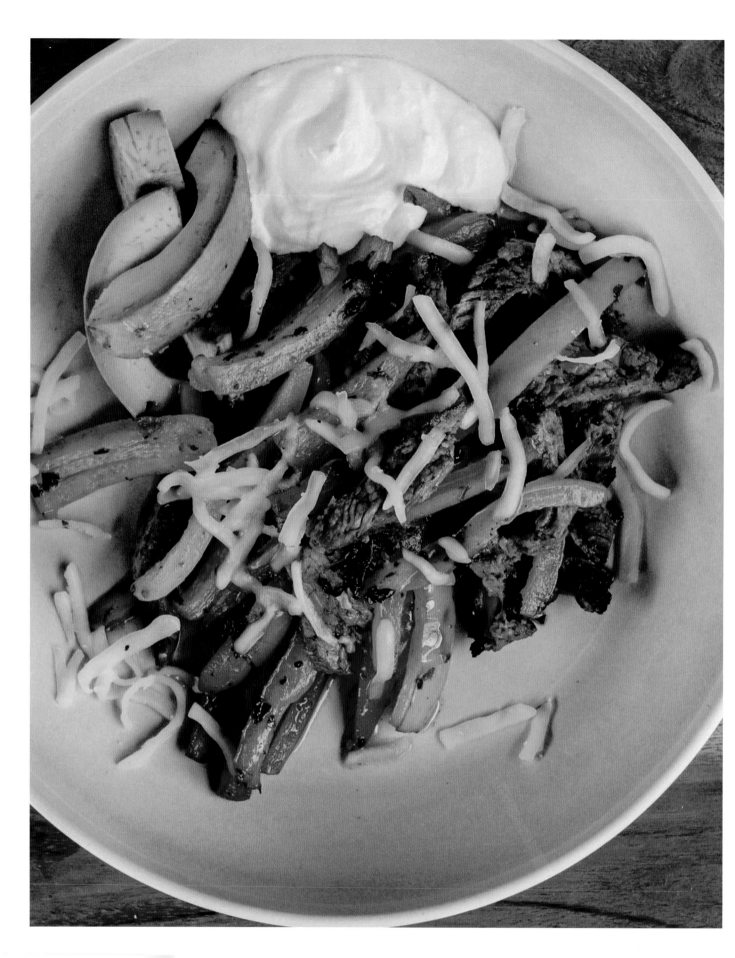

CHILI-LIME STEAK FAJITAS

Fire up your cast-iron skillet for this fast and easy recipe and get ready to dig in! If you have a food processor or blender, you can blend the marinade ingredients in it. Enjoy this dish as is, or serve with a side of leafy greens, riced cauliflower, or low-carb tortillas.

MARINADE:

- 2 **tablespoons (30 mL) extra-virgin olive oil**
- 2 **tablespoons (30 mL) fresh lime juice**
- 2 **garlic cloves, minced**
- 1 **teaspoon (5 g) sea salt**
- ½ **teaspoon (1 g) black pepper**
- 2 **teaspoons (10 g) ground cumin**
- 1 **teaspoon (5 g) red pepper flakes**
- 1 **bunch fresh cilantro leaves, minced**

FAJITAS:

- 6 **ounces (170 g) flank steak**
- 2 **medium (300 g) bell peppers (any color), seeded and sliced**

GARNISH:

- 1 **medium (150 g) avocado, peeled, pitted, and sliced**
- 2 **tablespoons (30 g) full-fat sour cream**
- ¼ **cup (28 g) shredded mozzarella cheese**

INSTRUCTIONS:

Combine all the marinade ingredients in a shallow dish and whisk to mix well. Add the flank steak, tossing until the steak is coated. Allow to marinate for 15 minutes.

Heat a cast-iron skillet over medium heat. When hot, add the flank steak and cook to your desired doneness, 3–5 minutes per side. Transfer the steak to a plate. When cool enough to handle, slice into thin strips.

Add the bell peppers to the skillet and sauté until soft, about 5 minutes. Transfer the peppers to the plate with the steak. Serve topped with the avocado, sour cream, and mozzarella cheese.

SERVES **2**
PREP TIME: **15 MINUTES**
COOKING TIME: **15 MINUTES**

CALORIES: **483**
CARBS: **12**
PROTEIN: **25**
FAT: **37**

SLOW COOKER STEAK FAJITAS

Let this recipe cook all day in your slow cooker and get ready for a mouthwatering meal when it's ready. Serve over a bed of riced cauliflower and increase its healthy fats by serving with full-fat sour cream or sliced avocado.

- 2 **tablespoons (30 g) butter, melted**
- 1 **teaspoon (5 g) sea salt**
- ½ **teaspoon (1 g) black pepper**
- 1 **teaspoon (5 g) red pepper flakes**
- 2 **tablespoons (30 g) chili powder**
- 3 **garlic cloves, minced**
- 2 **cups (480 mL) marinara sauce**
- 1 **pound (454 g) flank or ribeye steak, sliced against the grain**
- 1 **medium (150 g) yellow onion, sliced**
- 2 **medium (150 g) bell peppers, seeded and sliced**
- ¼ **cup (16 g) chopped fresh cilantro, for garnish**

INSTRUCTIONS:

Combine the melted butter, sea salt, black pepper, red pepper flakes, chili powder, and minced garlic in a slow cooker and stir well. Stir in the marinara sauce. Add the sliced steak, onion, and bell peppers and gently toss to combine.

Cover and cook on low for 8 hours or on high for 4 hours. Serve hot, garnished with fresh cilantro. Store leftovers in an airtight container in the fridge for up to 3 days.

SERVES 4
PREP TIME: 10 MINUTES
COOKING TIME: 4–8 HOURS

CALORIES: 588
CARBS: 24
PROTEIN: 52
FAT: 31

CLASSIC BEEF STEW

This traditional stew is keto-friendly, made with melt-in-your-mouth chunks of beef and lots of fresh veggies. This dish can also be slow-cooked or pressure-cooked, so don't skip making it if you're not able to be home while it simmers on the stove.

- 1 pound (454 g) beef chuck roast, cubed
- 2 teaspoons (10 g) sea salt, divided
- 1 teaspoon (2 g) black pepper, divided
- 4 tablespoons (60 g) butter, plus more if needed, divided
- 1 cup (100 g) sliced cremini mushrooms
- 1 medium (150 g) yellow onion, diced
- 1 medium (50 g) carrot, peeled and diced
- 2 medium (100 g) celery stalks, chopped
- 3 garlic cloves
- 2 tablespoons (30 g) tomato paste
- 2 cups (480 mL) beef stock
- 1 teaspoon (5 g) dried thyme
- 1 teaspoon (5 g) dried rosemary
- Minced fresh parsley, for garnish

INSTRUCTIONS:

Pat the beef dry with paper towels and season with 1 teaspoon of the sea salt and ½ teaspoon of the black pepper. Melt 2 tablespoons of the butter in a large pot over medium heat. Working in batches, add the beef and sear until golden all over, about 3 minutes per side. As each batch browns, transfer to a plate and continue with the remaining beef, adding more butter as necessary.

Add the mushrooms to the pot and cook until golden and crispy, about 5 minutes. Add the onion, carrot, and celery and cook until soft, about 5 minutes. Add the garlic and cook until fragrant, 1 minute more. Add the tomato paste and remaining 2 tablespoons of butter and stir to coat the vegetables.

Add the stock, thyme, rosemary, and beef to the pot and season with the remaining 1 teaspoon sea salt and remaining ½ teaspoon black pepper. Bring to a boil, then reduce the heat and simmer until the beef is tender, 50 minutes to 1 hour. Serve garnished with fresh parsley.

SERVES 4	CALORIES: 410
PREP TIME: 15 MINUTES	CARBS: 10
COOKING TIME: 1½ HOURS	PROTEIN: 32
	FAT: 30

ORGAN
MEAT
ENTREES

Organs were a centerpiece of the ancestral human diet and are widely regarded as the most nutrient-dense foods on earth. They remain a fixture in many traditional cuisines around the world but have been egregiously neglected in the fast-food era. These preparations will help you reconnect with your ancestral past and replenish depleted cellular energy with true superfood meals.

SWEET AND SAVORY CHICKEN LIVER BITES

If we had known that it was possible to sweeten up organ meats and still create optimal health, we would have been doing this a long time ago!

1 tablespoon (10 g) erythritol

1 teaspoon (2.5 g) smoked paprika

½ teaspoon (1.25 g) cayenne pepper

Sea salt and black pepper to taste

12 ounces (340 g) chicken livers

2 tablespoons (14 g) bacon bits

INSTRUCTIONS:

Combine the erythritol, smoked paprika, cayenne, sea salt, and black pepper in a zip-top bag. Add the chicken livers, seal the bag, and shake to coat the livers in the seasoning.

Heat a cast-iron skillet over medium heat. When hot, add the seasoned chicken livers and sear for 3–4 minutes per side. Garnish with the bacon bits and serve.

SERVES 2
PREP TIME: 5 MINUTES
COOKING TIME: 10 MINUTES

CALORIES: 618
CARBS: 3
PROTEIN: 55
FAT: 42

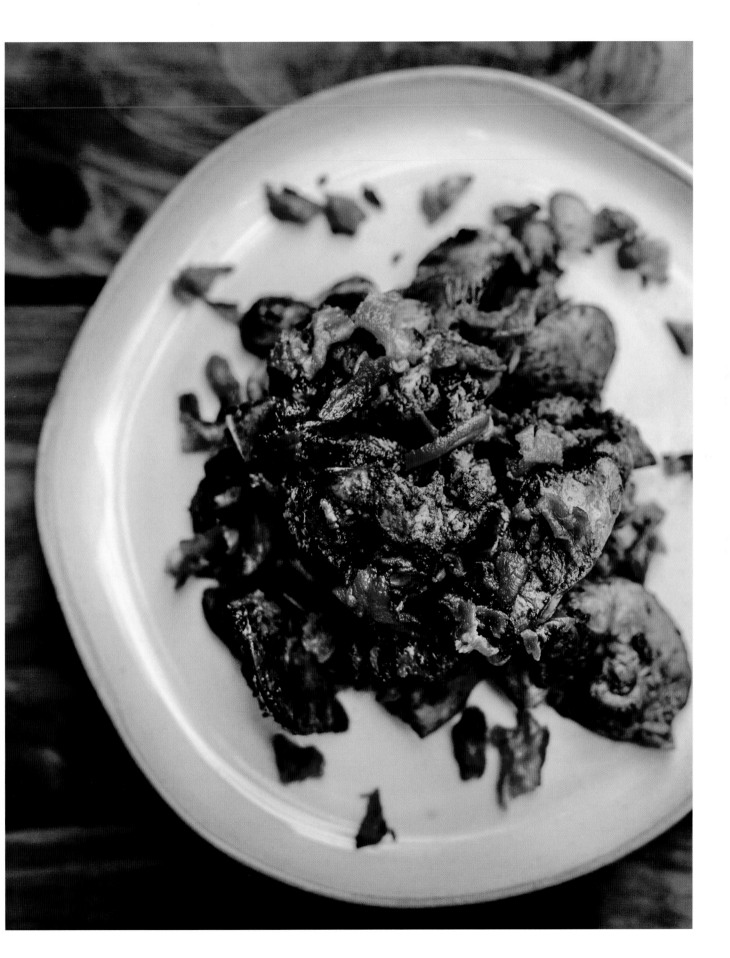

SIMPLE LIVER PÂTÉ

You only need a few ingredients for this delicious pâté recipe. Liver, bacon grease, and thyme are combined with creamy coconut and savory onion and garlic in this recipe. Enjoy on its own or with veggie crudités.

1 **tablespoon (15 g) bacon fat**

1 **tablespoon (4 g) minced red onion**

1 **garlic clove, minced**

4 **ounces (114 g) beef liver, chopped**

½ **teaspoon (2.5 g) sea salt**

½ **teaspoon (1 g) black pepper**

1 **teaspoon (2.5 g) dried thyme**

1 **tablespoon (15 g) canned coconut cream**

¼ **cup (60 mL) purified water**

INSTRUCTIONS:

Melt the bacon fat in a skillet over medium heat. Add the onion and garlic and sauté until browned and soft, about 5 minutes. Add the liver, season with the sea salt, black pepper, and thyme, and sauté until the liver is brown on the outside but still pink on the inside, about 5 minutes per side.

Transfer the contents of the skillet to a food processor. Add the coconut cream and purified water and process until very smooth. Transfer to a serving bowl and serve.

SERVES 8

PREP TIME: 10 MINUTES

COOKING TIME: 15 MINUTES

CALORIES: 114

CARBS: 0

PROTEIN: 4

FAT: 9

HEART AND KIDNEY STEW

Your slow cooker is your best friend for this recipe—just load it up with the ingredients, set it, and go about your day and you'll have a delicious bowl of stew ready when you are. Organ meats steal the show in this recipe. If you can't find chicken hearts, just use beef.

2   **pounds (912 g) chicken hearts**

1   **pound (454 g) beef kidney**

1   **medium (150 g) yellow onion, chopped**

3   **garlic cloves, minced**

1   **medium head (560 g) cauliflower, chopped**

1   **cup (75 g) chopped cremini mushrooms**

1   **tablespoon (7 g) dried oregano**

1   **teaspoon (1.25 g) dried rosemary**

1   **tablespoon (15 g) sea salt**

2   **teaspoons (4 g) black pepper**

6   **cups (1140 mL) chicken or beef bone broth**

Chopped fresh parsley, for garnish

INSTRUCTIONS:

Combine all the ingredients in a slow cooker, cover, and cook on low for 4 hours. Garnish with fresh parsley and serve.

SERVES **8**

PREP TIME: **10 MINUTES**

COOKING TIME: **4 HOURS**

CALORIES: **328**

CARBS: **7**

PROTEIN: **44**

FAT: **13**

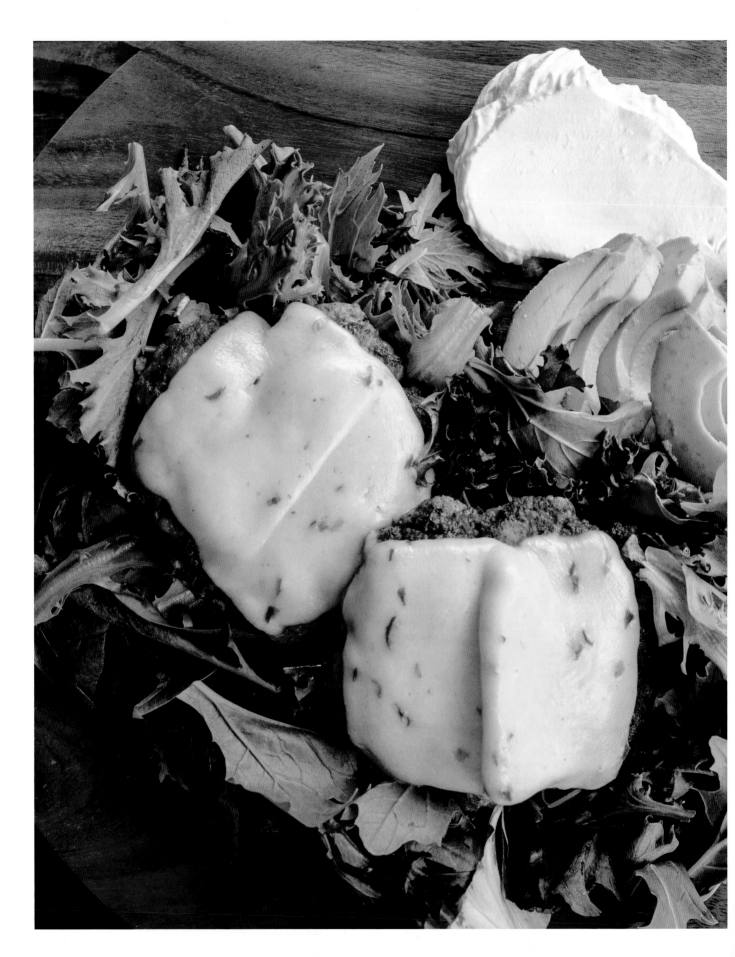

ORGAN MEAT BURGERS

Burgers are the perfect way to introduce more organ meats into your diet. Start by adding liver or heart or try this recipe, which includes beef spleen. Serve with all your favorite burger condiments.

1 **pound (454 g) ground beef**

4 **ounces (114 g) beef spleen, minced**

4 **ounces (114 g) beef kidney, minced**

2 **thin bacon strips (or 1 thick strip), chopped into small bits**

3 **garlic cloves, minced**

Handful fresh parsley leaves, chopped

1 **tablespoon (7 g) dried oregano**

1 **teaspoon (1.25 g) dried rosemary**

1 **tablespoon (15 g) sea salt**

2 **teaspoons (4 g) black pepper**

1 **tablespoon (15 g) bacon grease, butter, or beef tallow**

4 **ounces (114 g) pepper Jack cheese, sliced**

GARNISH:

Avocado, sliced (optional)

Mixed greens (optional)

Cream cheese, or similar soft cheese (optional)

INSTRUCTIONS:

Combine all the ingredients except the bacon grease in a large bowl and use your hands to form into 4 patties.

Heat the bacon grease in a cast-iron skillet over medium-high heat. Add the patties and cook to your preferred doneness, about 3 minutes per side for medium-rare. Place pepper Jack cheese slices on top of the patties until lightly melted. Serve with garnishes as desired.

SERVES 4
PREP TIME: 10 MINUTES
COOKING TIME: 15 MINUTES

CALORIES: 469
CARBS: 2
PROTEIN: 48
FAT: 29

CHICKEN HEARTS AND LEEKS

This recipe, inspired by simple French cuisine, will nourish your body. Always remember how good you feel when you choose basic proteins such as chicken hearts and flavor-enhancing veggies such as leeks.

2 **tablespoons (30 g) butter**

2 **medium (30 g) leeks, trimmed and chopped**

3 **garlic cloves, minced**

1 **teaspoon (5 g) sea salt**

½ **teaspoon (1 g) black pepper**

1 **pound (454 g) chicken hearts**

Minced fresh parsley, for garnish

INSTRUCTIONS:

Melt the butter in a skillet over medium heat. Add the leeks and garlic, season with the sea salt and black pepper, and sauté until soft and browned, about 5 minutes.

Push the leeks to one side of the skillet, add the chicken hearts, and cook until browned, about 1 minute per side. Garnish with fresh parsley and serve.

SERVES 4

PREP TIME: **10 MINUTES**

COOKING TIME: **10 MINUTES**

CALORIES: 229

CARBS: 3

PROTEIN: 17

FAT: 16

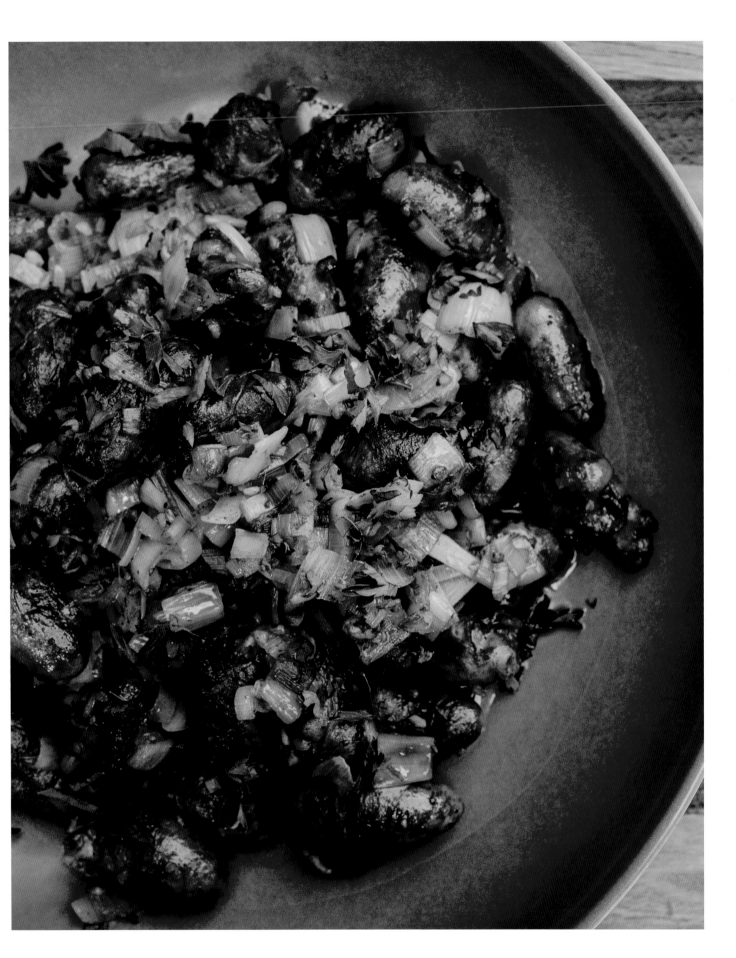

CHICKEN LIVERS WITH HERBED YOGURT SAUCE

This dish is wonderful on its own or served over a bed of mixed salad greens for some extra crunch. Full-fat Greek yogurt is super satisfying—you won't want to settle for fat-free after you try it!

YOGURT SAUCE:

- 2 cups (570 g) full-fat Greek yogurt
- 1 teaspoon (5 g) sea salt
- ½ teaspoon (1 g) black pepper
- Handful fresh parsley leaves, minced
- 1 scallion, minced
- Grated zest of ½ lemon

CHICKEN LIVERS:

- 2 tablespoons (30 g) butter
- 1 pound (454 g) chicken livers, chopped
- 3 garlic cloves, minced
- 1 teaspoon (5 g) sea salt
- ½ teaspoon (1 g) black pepper

INSTRUCTIONS:

Combine all the yogurt sauce ingredients in a medium bowl and mix well. Set aside until ready to serve.

Melt the butter in a skillet over medium heat. Add the livers and garlic, season with the sea salt and black pepper, and sauté until soft and browned, about 5 minutes. Serve the livers with the yogurt sauce.

SERVES 4
PREP TIME: 10 MINUTES
COOKING TIME: 5 MINUTES

CALORIES: 294
CARBS: 6
PROTEIN: 0
FAT: 15

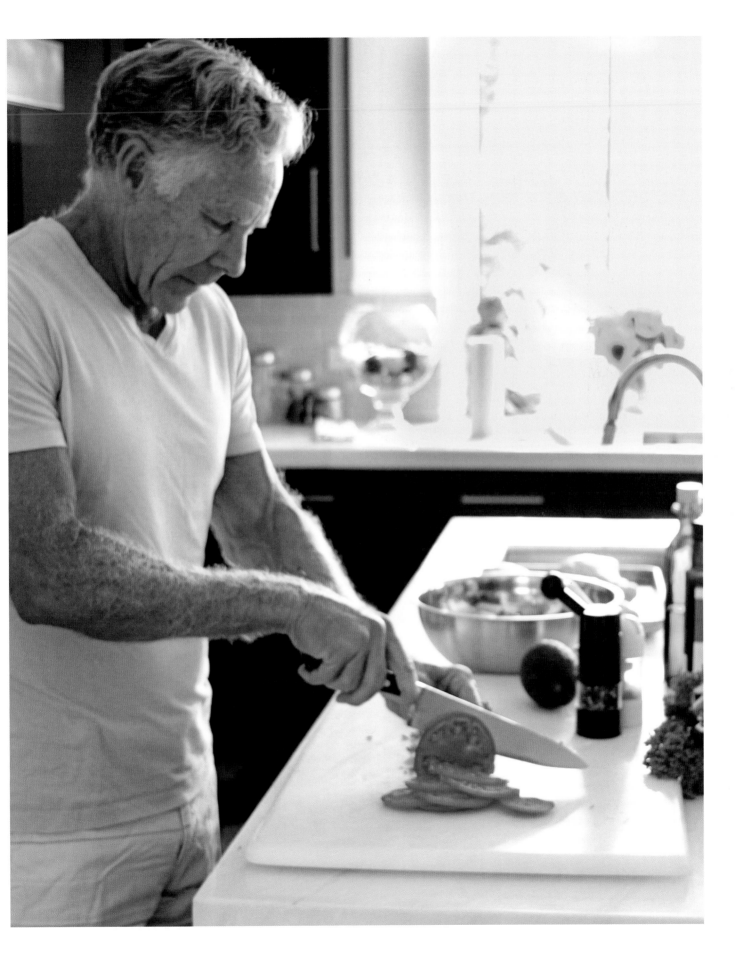

CARNI-VORE-ISH ENTREES

CHAPTER 9

These recipes will boost the nutrient density of your diet, provide an incredible level of satiety, and also allow you to perform a plant food restriction experiment in hopes of improving nagging inflammatory or autoimmune conditions. A carnivore-ish strategy has also shown to be effective for fat reduction. You will consume minimal carbohydrates but feel totally satisfied after each meal.

BLUE CHEESE BUFFALO BURGERS

This one takes the cake (...or steak?) for my absolute favorite carnivore meal. Blue cheese and buffalo—you can't go wrong.

- 2 **pounds (908 g) ground bison**
- 2 **teaspoons (10 g) Himalayan pink salt**
- 1 **teaspoon (2 g) black pepper**
- ½ **cup (230 g) crumbled blue cheese, divided into 8 tablespoons**
- **Mixed greens, for serving**

INSTRUCTIONS:

Season the ground bison with the pink salt and pepper. Form the ground bison into 4 balls. Poke a hole in each ball and press 1 tablespoon blue cheese into the hole. Seal the meat around the cheese. Press the balls into patties.

Pan-fry the burgers in a skillet over medium heat until done to your liking, 4–6 minutes per side. Garnish each cooked patty with 1 tablespoon blue cheese.

Serve on a bed of mixed greens.

SERVES 4
PREP TIME: **10 MINUTES**
COOKING TIME: **10 MINUTES**

CALORIES: **464**
CARBS: **1**
PROTEIN: **31**
FAT: **45**

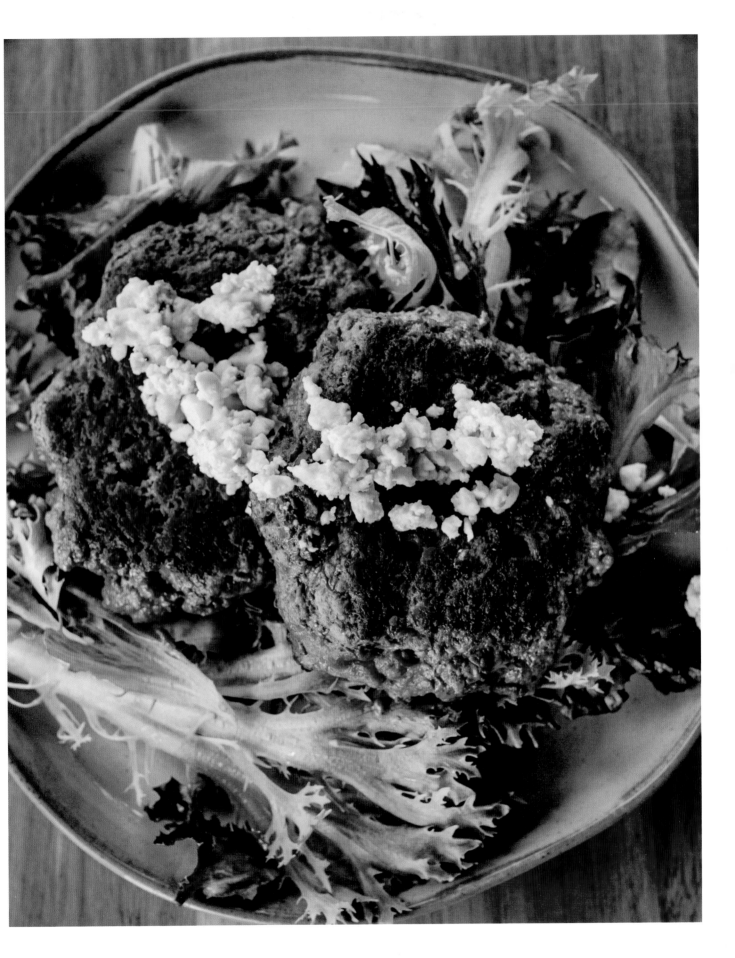

NUT BUTTER GROUND BEEF

Macadamia and cashew nut butter are solid choices for those looking to minimize oxalates.

1 **pound (454 g) lean ground beef**

2 **tablespoons (32 g) macadamia or cashew butter**

20 **g (1–2 scoops) unflavored collagen peptides (Primal Kitchen or Vital Proteins)**

INSTRUCTIONS:

Heat a skillet over medium-high heat. When hot, brown the ground beef, breaking up the meat until cooked through, 5–7 minutes. Mix in the nut butter and collagen peptides and serve.

SERVES 4
PREP TIME: **10 MINUTES**
COOKING TIME: **10 MINUTES**

CALORIES: **295**
CARBS: **1**
PROTEIN: **27**
FAT: **21**

COTTAGE CHEESE PROTEIN BOMB

Sometimes being a carnivore on the go can be a little tough, so here's a cheap and easy snack that will keep you full and nourished!

1 (4.4-ounce/125 g) can sardines, packed in water, drained

2 cups (324 g) cottage cheese

2 tablespoons (14 g) bacon bits

INSTRUCTIONS:

Combine all the ingredients in a bowl and enjoy!

SERVES 1
PREP TIME: 5 MINUTES

CALORIES: 685
CARBS: 20
PROTEIN: 83
FAT: 33

CHICKEN HEART SKEWERS

These skewers are a Mediterranean classic. You get all of the amazing nutrients of chicken hearts with a nice kick from ground cumin.

1 **pound (454 g) chicken hearts**

1 **teaspoon (5 g) sea salt**

¼ **teaspoon (0.5 g) black pepper**

⅛ **teaspoon (0.3 g) cayenne pepper**

1 **teaspoon (2.5 g) ground cumin**

Fresh parsley leaves, for garnish

INSTRUCTIONS:

Heat the grill to medium-high heat. Thread the chicken hearts onto skewers. Season with the sea salt, black pepper, cayenne, and cumin. Grill until firm throughout, about 10–15 minutes. Garnish with parsley and serve.

SERVES 4
PREP TIME: 5 MINUTES
COOKING TIME: 15 MINUTES

CALORIES: 176
CARBS: 1
PROTEIN: 18
FAT: 11

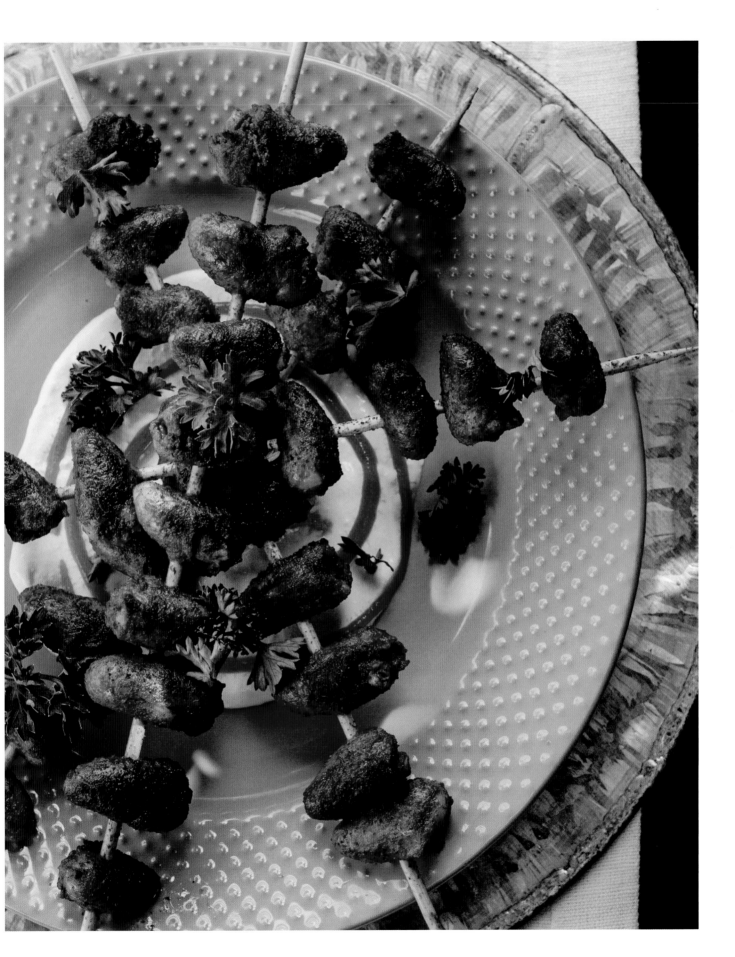

SLOW-COOKED BACON-WRAPPED MEATLOAF

This is a perfect dish to create for friends and family at a special gathering—just prep it and let it cook in your slow cooker!

1½   pounds (681 g) ground beef

1   medium (150 g) yellow onion, chopped

2   garlic cloves, minced

1   cup (30 g) baby spinach

1   medium (150 g) bell pepper (any color), seeded and chopped

½   cup (50 g) almond flour

1   large egg, whisked

1   teaspoon (5 mL) Worcestershire sauce

1   teaspoon (5 g) sea salt

1   teaspoon (2 g) black pepper

1   pound (454 g) bacon strips

INSTRUCTIONS:

In a large bowl, mix together all the ingredients except the bacon.

Lay a large sheet of parchment paper flat on the counter. Lay out the uncooked bacon, perfectly connected, on the parchment paper. Place the meatloaf mixture in the center of the bacon lineup and form into a meatloaf shape. Carefully wrap the meatloaf with the bacon strips. Place the meatloaf in a slow cooker, cover, and cook on high for 4–5 hours or on low for 6–8 hours.

Preheat the broiler. Drain the liquid from the slow cooker. Place the slow cooker insert under the broiler for a few minutes to crisp up the bacon.

SERVES 8
PREP TIME: 10 MINUTES
COOKING TIME: 4–8 HOURS

CALORIES: 544
CARBS: 5
PROTEIN: 26
FAT: 46

MEAT MUFFINS

These are a cinch to prepare and pop in your mouth so easily, you'll love being able to grab them on the go! Flavor with your favorite dried spices and herbs and play around with different cheeses such as feta or goat.

1½ pounds (681 g) ground beef

1 medium (150 g) yellow onion, diced

1 large egg, whisked

1 teaspoon (5 g) sea salt

1 teaspoon (2 g) black pepper

1 cup (114 g) shredded extra-sharp Cheddar cheese

INSTRUCTIONS:

Preheat the oven to 350°F (180°C).

In a large bowl, combine the ground beef, onion, egg, sea salt, and black pepper. Mix the ingredients together with your hands and gently place a small handful of the mixture into each cup of a 12-cup muffin tin. Top with the grated cheese. Bake until cooked through, 15–20 minutes. Allow to cool for a few minutes before serving.

SERVES 12

PREP TIME: 10 MINUTES

COOKING TIME: 20 MINUTES

CALORIES: 221

CARBS: 1

PROTEIN: 15

FAT: 17

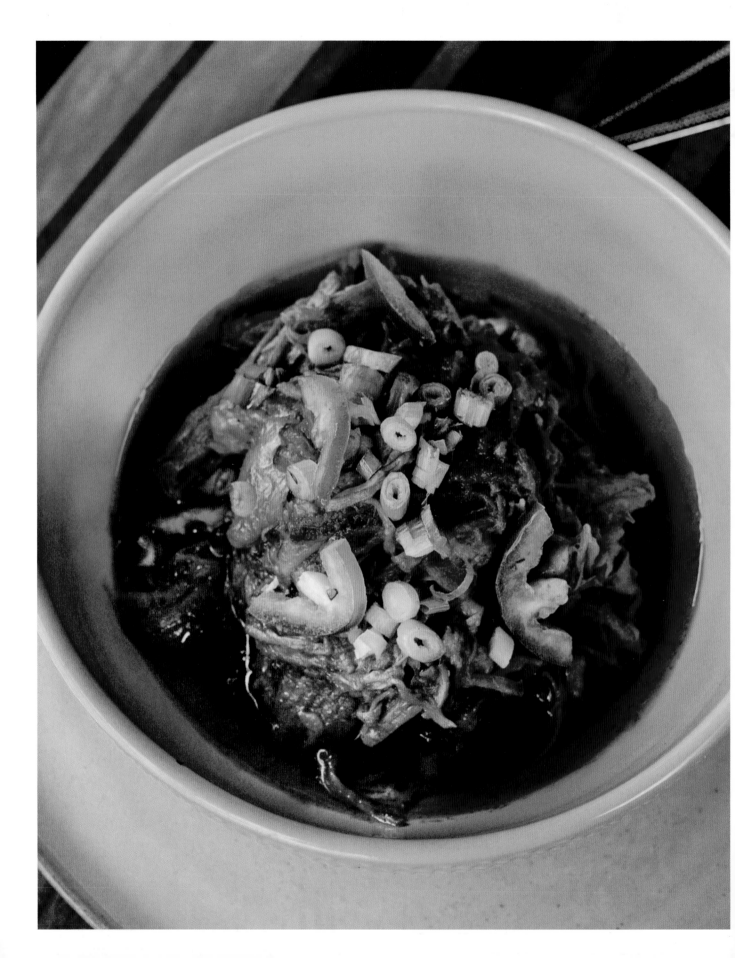

SLOW-COOKED PULLED PORK

This tastes amazing right out of the slow cooker—no sugary BBQ sauce is needed!

1 tablespoon (15 g) tomato paste

1 tablespoon (15 mL) coconut aminos

1 teaspoon (5 g) ground cumin

1 teaspoon (5 g) smoked paprika

1 teaspoon (5 g) sea salt

1 teaspoon (2 g) black pepper

1 tablespoon (15 g) onion powder

1 tablespoon (3.75 g) garlic powder

1¾ pounds (800 g) pork shoulder

¼ cup (60 mL) raw apple cider vinegar

GARNISH:

Sliced jalapeño

Sliced scallion

INSTRUCTIONS:

In a slow cooker, whisk together the tomato paste, coconut aminos, and all the seasonings. Place the pork shoulder in the slow cooker, skin side down, and completely rub it all over with the seasoned paste.

Flip the roast so that the skin side is facing up. Add the vinegar to the slow cooker by pouring it to the side, not over the roast. Cover and cook on low for 10–12 hours or on high for 8 hours.

When done, shred the roast and return the meat to the slow cooker to rest and absorb the juices for 10–15 minutes. Garnish with sliced jalapeño and scallion and serve.

SERVES 8
PREP TIME: 10 MINUTES
COOKING TIME: 8–12 HOURS

CALORIES: 181
CARBS: 1
PROTEIN: 25
FAT: 8

CHEESE AND CHICKEN MEATBALLS

Eat these meatballs as a snack or as your next favorite carnivore meal! We love 'em served with a side of mayo.

- 1 **medium (150 g) yellow onion**
- 4 **garlic cloves, peeled**
- 2¼ **pounds (568 g) ground chicken**
- 4 **large eggs**
- 1 **cup (114 g) shredded mozzarella cheese**
- 1 **cup (100 g) almond flour**
- 2 **teaspoons (10 g) sea salt**
- 1 **teaspoon (2 g) black pepper**

INSTRUCTIONS:

Preheat the oven to 350°F (180°C). Line a rimmed baking sheet with parchment paper.

Put the onion and garlic in a food processor and pulse until finely chopped. Add the remaining ingredients and pulse until completely combined.

Scoop out a portion of the cheesy chicken mixture about the size of a golf ball (approximately 1.5 inches in diameter) and roll or squeeze it into a ball. Place on the prepared baking sheet. Continue to make the remaining meatballs until the mixture is complete.

Bake until golden brown and cooked through, about 20 minutes. Allow to cool for a few minutes before serving.

SERVES 6
PREP TIME: **10 MINUTES**
COOKING TIME: **20 MINUTES**

CALORIES: **181**
CARBS: **1**
PROTEIN: **25**
FAT: **8**

CANNED SALMON EGG BAKE

This recipe uses staples from your kitchen—canned salmon, eggs, and butter. It's so easy, you don't even need dishes for this one. Just grab a fork and dig in.

1 (6-ounce/170 g) can salmon

1½ teaspoons (7 g) butter

1 large egg

INSTRUCTIONS:

Preheat the broiler or toaster oven.

Remove the salmon from the can and line the inside of the can with aluminum foil. Return the salmon to the can. Top with the butter, then crack the egg on top.

Broil or toast the can until the egg white is crispy and the yolk is slightly runny, about 15-20 minutes.

SERVES 1
PREP TIME: 5 MINUTES
COOKING TIME: 20 MINUTES

CALORIES: 427
CARBS: 0
PROTEIN: 72
FAT: 16

TUNA PATTIES

Adding collagen to this recipe makes these tuna patties even more nutritious. Make sure you always have some in your pantry and discover all the ways to sneak it into meals.

1 **large egg**

2 **(5-ounce/142 g) cans tuna, drained**

2 **tablespoons (18 g) unflavored hydrolysate collagen**

1 **tablespoon (15 mL) water**

1 **tablespoon (15 g) yellow mustard**

1 **teaspoon (5 g) sea salt**

1 **tablespoon (15 g) beef tallow**

Mixed greens, for serving

Lemon wedges, for garnish

INSTRUCTIONS:

In a medium bowl, beat the egg. Add the tuna, collagen, water, mustard, and sea salt. Form the mixture into 2 patties and let chill in the fridge for 1 hour.

Heat the tallow in a skillet over medium-high heat. Add the patties and cook until brown, 3–4 minutes per side. Serve over mixed greens and garnish with lemon wedges.

SERVES 2
PREP TIME: 10 MINUTES
COOKING TIME: 10 MINUTES

CALORIES: 353
CARBS: 1
PROTEIN: 41
FAT: 18

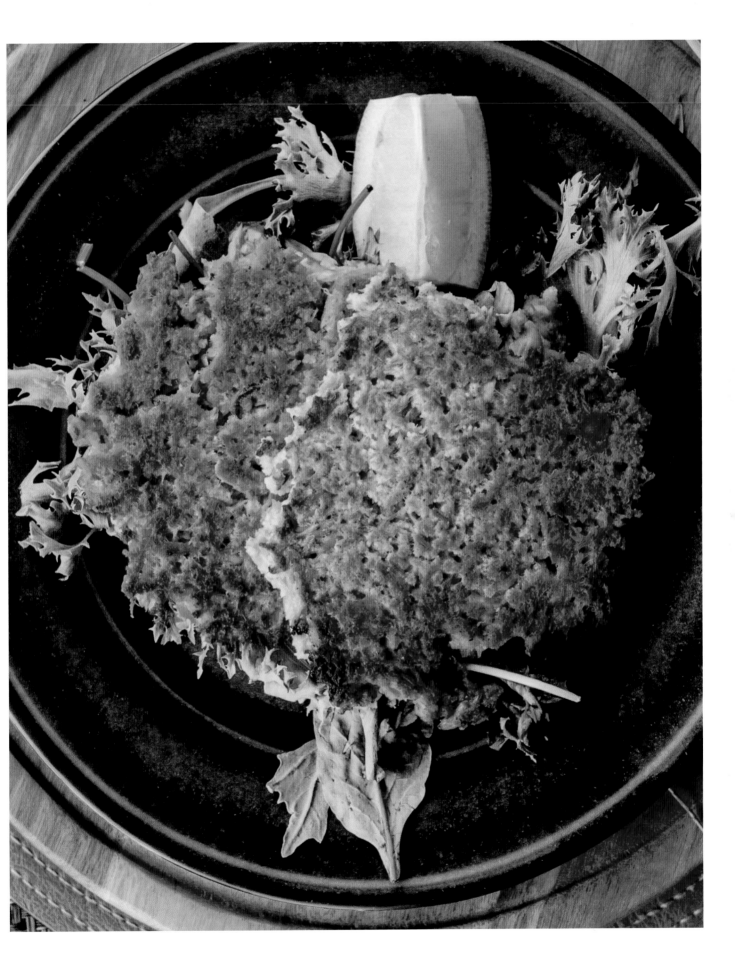

VENISON AND SALMON ROE

All right, enough steak and eggs. Let's get real and primal here. Ancient people weren't just hunting down cows all day, they were hunting down deer as well. Combine that with some salmon roe and you've got a serious nutritional-powerhouse meal.

- **2 teaspoons (10 g) beef tallow**
- **8 ounces (228 g) wild venison**
- **1 teaspoon (5 g) sea salt**
- **2 ounces (57 g) red salmon roe**

INSTRUCTIONS:

Melt the beef tallow in a skillet over medium heat. Season both sides of the venison with the sea salt and cook until cooked through, about 5 minutes per side. Top with the salmon roe and serve.

SERVES **1**

PREP TIME: **10 MINUTES**

COOKING TIME: **10 MINUTES**

CALORIES: **611**

CARBS: **0**

PROTEIN: **89**

FAT: **28**

GRASS-FED CHUCK ROAST

It doesn't get any easier than this. Just turn on your slow cooker, go about your day, and sit down to a hearty dinner later.

2 pounds (908 g) chuck roast

1 teaspoon (5 g) sea salt

INSTRUCTIONS:

Season the chuck roast all over with the sea salt. Put the roast in a slow cooker, cover, and cook on low for 5–8 hours.

SERVES 8
PREP TIME: 5 MINUTES
COOKING TIME: 5–8 HOURS

CALORIES: 253
CARBS: 0
PROTEIN: 28
FAT: 18

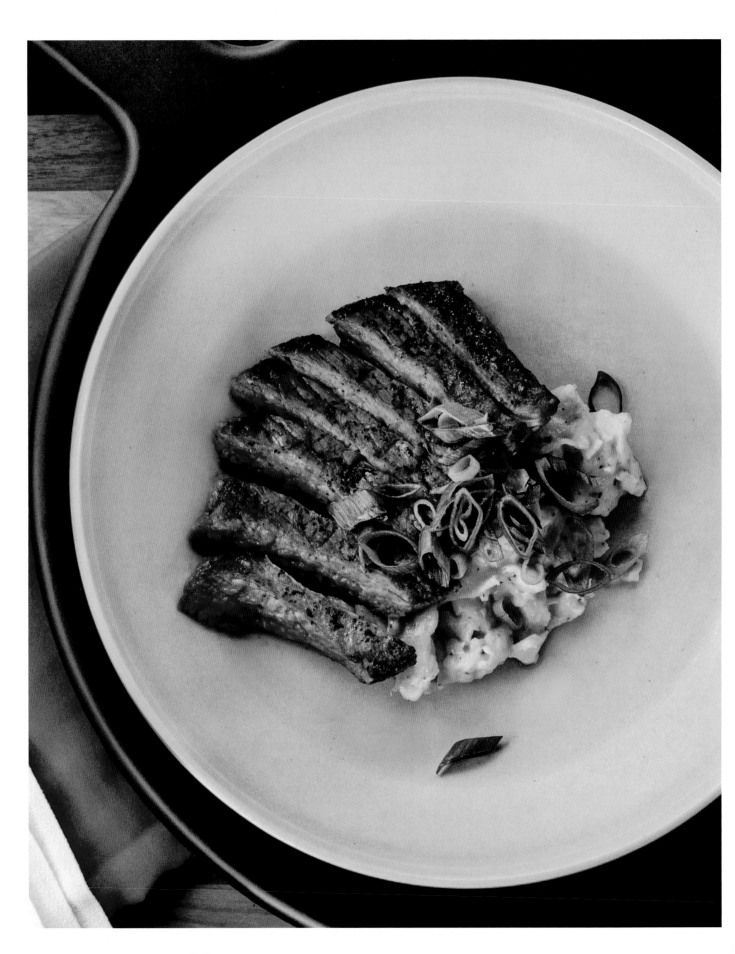

EXPRESS STEAK AND EGGS

Here's a steak-and-eggs recipe for when you're in a hurry. Microwaved eggs are actually pretty decent if you use a bit of bone broth and a bit of practice.

- 1 **tablespoon (15 g) beef tallow**

- 4 **ounces (114 g) top sirloin or other lean steak**

- 1 **teaspoon (5 g) sea salt**

- 2 **tablespoons (30 mL) bone broth**

- 2 **large eggs**

  Sliced scallions, for garnish

INSTRUCTIONS:

Heat the beef tallow in a cast-iron skillet over medium-high heat. Season the steak with the sea salt. When the pan is hot and almost smoking, add the steak and cook to your preferred doneness, 3–4 minutes per side. Let the steak rest for a minute or two.

While the steak is cooking, pour the bone broth into a mug. Microwave the mug for 45 seconds. Crack the eggs into the mug, whisk into the broth, and microwave for another 45 seconds. Slice and serve the steak with the eggs and scallions for garnish.

SERVES **1**

PREP TIME: **10 MINUTES**

COOKING TIME: **10 MINUTES**

CALORIES: **406**

CARBS: **5**

PROTEIN: **60**

FAT: **15**

SEARED LAMB CHOPS

Beef ain't the only red meat! Switch things up and try some of these delicious lamb chops.

8 ounces (226 g) lamb chops

Sea salt and black pepper to taste

1 tablespoon (15 mL) extra-virgin olive oil

INSTRUCTIONS:

Preheat the oven to 400°F (200°C).

Pat the lamb chops dry with a paper towel, then season generously with sea salt and black pepper.

Heat the olive oil in a skillet over medium-high heat until smoking. Add the lamb chops and cook until a golden-brown crust forms on the bottom, about 3 minutes. Flip and cook until the second side is golden brown, another 3 minutes.

Transfer the lamb chops to a rimmed baking sheet and roast until cooked through, 8–10 minutes. Let rest for 5 minutes before serving.

SERVES 1
PREP TIME: 5 MINUTES
COOKING TIME: 15 MINUTES

CALORIES: 298
CARBS: 0
PROTEIN: 27
FAT: 23

BACON AND LIVER

You know liver's good for you. And you could be experiencing the superhuman benefits of the carnivore diet if only you could stop gagging at the thought of liver. We gotcha. By quickly searing liver in bacon fat, you get all the delicious flavor of bacon on the liver. You also avoid overcooking the liver, which leads to the chalky taste and consistency people hate.

5 **bacon strips**

4 **ounces (114 g) calf liver**

INSTRUCTIONS:

Cook the bacon in a skillet over medium heat until crispy, 5–7 minutes. Transfer the bacon to a plate, leaving the bacon grease in the skillet.

Add the liver to the skillet and sear for 20 seconds on each side. Place the liver on top of the bacon and serve.

SERVES **1**

PREP TIME: **5 MINUTES**

COOKING TIME: **10 MINUTES**

CALORIES: **415**

CARBS: **4**

PROTEIN: **45**

FAT: **25**

CHEESE CRISPS AND LIVER PÂTÉ

Cheese crisps are the ultimate carnivore hack if you need some crunch in your life. Combine with liver pâté and you've got a formidable micronutrient punch!

1 tablespoon (15 g) butter

1 pound (454 g) beef livers, cut in half

½ cup (120 mL) beef broth

Sea salt and black pepper to taste

Cheese crisps, for serving

INSTRUCTIONS:

Melt the butter in a skillet over low heat. Add the liver and cook, stirring occasionally, until cooked through, 7–10 minutes.

Remove from the heat and cool slightly. Transfer the liver to a blender, add the broth, and puree until smooth. Season with sea salt and black pepper. Pour the pureed liver into a bowl or container and refrigerate until chilled. Serve with cheese crisps.

SERVES 4

PREP TIME: 10 MINUTES

COOKING TIME: 15 MINUTES

CALORIES: 194

CARBS: 4

PROTEIN: 25

FAT: 7

COTTAGE CHEESE AND TUNA SALAD

Here's another meal with a super-high protein-to-energy ratio to help you get shredded.

2 (5-ounce/114 g) cans tuna, drained

⅔ cup (108 g) low-fat cottage cheese

1 tablespoon (15 g) yellow mustard

1 tablespoon (15 mL) lemon juice

½ teaspoon (0.7 g) garlic powder (optional)

INSTRUCTIONS:

Combine all the ingredients in a bowl and dig in!

SERVES **1**
PREP TIME: **5 MINUTES**

CALORIES: **370**
CARBS: **10**
PROTEIN: **69**
FAT: **7**

BRAISED CHICKEN WITH LEMON

Lemon slices transform a dish with their bright and complex flavor, so we like to use them as often as possible. Keep lemons stocked in your fridge and add them to roasted veggies and meats—but be sure to toss their seeds, which, though tiny in size, pack an undesirable bitter flavor.

1 tablespoon (15 g) ghee or butter

1 medium (160 g) yellow onion, chopped

1 pound (454 g) boneless, skinless chicken thighs

1 teaspoon (5 g) sea salt

1 teaspoon (2 g) black pepper

1 teaspoon (1.25 g) garlic powder

1 (13.5-ounce/398 mL) can full-fat coconut milk

1 tablespoon (7 g) yellow curry powder

1 lemon slice, seeded and minced

Sliced scallions, for garnish

Chopped cashews, for garnish

INSTRUCTIONS:

Melt the ghee in a skillet or Dutch oven over medium-high heat. Add the onion and sauté until soft, about 5 minutes. Add the chicken thighs and sprinkle with the sea salt, black pepper, and garlic powder. Reduce the heat to a simmer and add the coconut milk, curry powder, and minced lemon and gently stir everything together. Simmer until the coconut milk has thickened and the chicken is very tender, about 30 minutes.

Serve topped with some sliced scallions and a handful of chopped cashews.

SERVES 4
PREP TIME: 10 MINUTES
COOKING TIME: 35 MINUTES

CALORIES: 421
CARBS: 7
PROTEIN: 32
FAT: 28

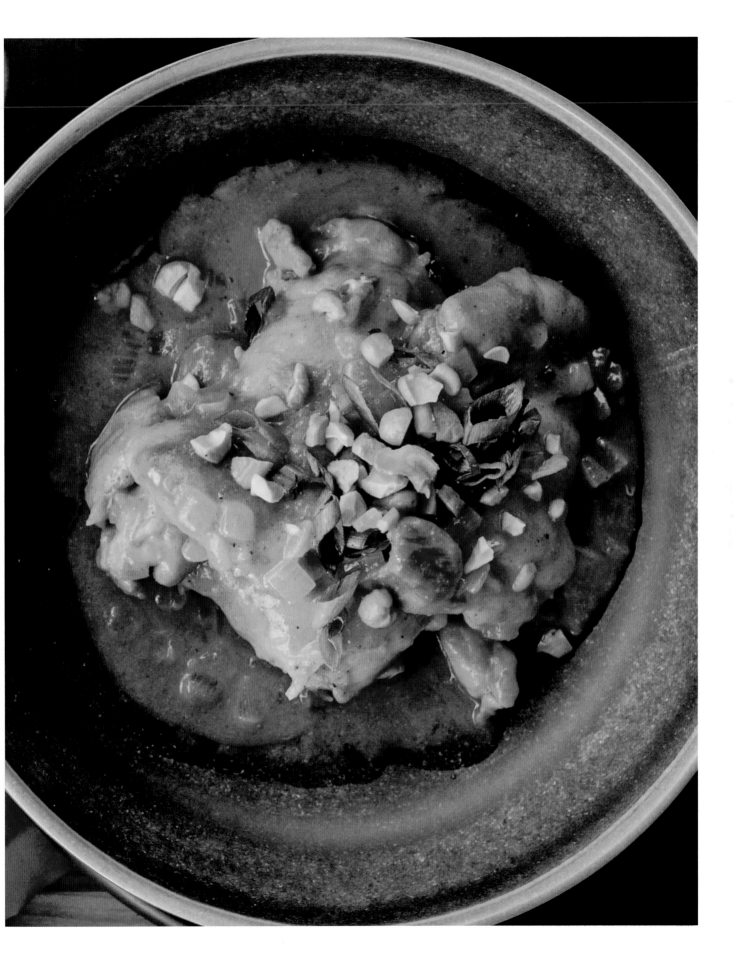

SEAFOOD ENTREES

CHAPTER 10

Don't forget about all the wonderful nutrients and healthy fats found in fish and shellfish! Not only are these recipes delicious but they are easy to make and don't require much time to prepare. You'll have more time to crush your goals and to-do list, so what are you waiting for?

SIMPLE SALMON AND ASPARAGUS

This delicious meal is amazing served with a side of roasted sweet potatoes or riced cauliflower, or over a big bed of wilted greens. Don't be afraid of cooking with lots of butter—your body loves its healthy fat!

- **4 tablespoons (60 g) butter**
- **1 pound (454 g) asparagus, trimmed and chopped**
- **4 garlic cloves, minced**
- **1 teaspoon (5 g) sea salt**
- **½ teaspoon (1 g) black pepper**
- **1 pound (454 g) salmon fillets**
- **½ cup (120 g) full-fat sour cream**
- **Grated zest of 1 lemon**

INSTRUCTIONS:

Melt the butter in a skillet over medium-low heat. Add the asparagus and garlic and sauté until the asparagus is soft and the garlic is golden, about 5 minutes. Season with the sea salt and black pepper and continue to sauté until soft, about 3 more minutes. Transfer the asparagus to a plate, reserving the butter in the skillet.

Increase the heat to medium-high. Place the salmon fillets in the skillet and sear without moving the fillets until just cooked through, 1–2 minutes per side.

Serve the salmon and asparagus, pouring the butter from the skillet over each dish and garnishing with a dollop of sour cream and zest of lemon. Store leftovers in an airtight container in the fridge for up to 3 days.

SERVES 4
PREP TIME: 5 MINUTES
COOKING TIME: 15 MINUTES

CALORIES: 380
CARBS: 6
PROTEIN: 36
FAT: 24

SALMON IN CREAMY CAPER SAUCE

This recipe will have you swooning for a dinner that is elegant yet so simple to prepare. If you don't have salmon, other good choices are shrimp, scallops, or white fish.

- 2 **tablespoons (30 g) butter**
- 2 **garlic cloves, minced**
- 1 **cup (240 mL) heavy cream**
- 1 **teaspoon (5 g) sea salt**
- ½ **teaspoon (1 g) black pepper**
- 2 **tablespoons (30 g) capers**
- **Grated zest of ½ lemon**
- 1 **pound (454 g) wild-caught salmon fillets, cut into bite-size pieces**
- **Minced fresh parsley, for garnish**

INSTRUCTIONS:

Melt the butter in a skillet over medium heat. Add the garlic and sauté until it begins to turn golden, about 3 minutes. Stir in the cream, sea salt, black pepper, capers, and lemon zest and reduce the heat to low. Add the salmon and simmer until the salmon has cooked through, about 3 more minutes. Top with fresh parsley and serve.

SERVES 4
PREP TIME: 5 MINUTES
COOKING TIME: 10 MINUTES

CALORIES: 503
CARBS: 5
PROTEIN: 32
FAT: 37

BAKED LEMON SALMON WITH GREEN BEANS

A simple dish gets extra special when fresh lemon slices are placed on top of wild-caught salmon fillets. Serve with a side of French green beans and some healthful mayonnaise for a delicious treat!

1 pound (454 g) French green beans

4 (6-ounce/170 g) wild-caught, skin-on salmon fillets

¼ cup (60 mL) extra-virgin olive oil

2 teaspoons (10 g) sea salt

1 teaspoon (2 g) black pepper

1 teaspoon (5 g) dried dill

4 lemon slices

GARNISH:

Minced fresh parsley

¼ cup (60 g) mayonnaise

INSTRUCTIONS:

Preheat the oven to 350°F (180°C). Line a rimmed baking sheet with parchment paper.

Spread out the green beans on the prepared baking sheet. Place the salmon fillets on top of the green beans. Brush the salmon with the olive oil and season with the sea salt, black pepper, and dill. Place a lemon slice on top of each fillet.

Bake until the salmon begins to flake and the lemon slices and green beans have softened, about 15 minutes. Garnish with minced parsley and top with a dollop of mayonnaise.

SERVES 4
PREP TIME: 10 MINUTES
COOKING TIME: 15 MINUTES

CALORIES: 604
CARBS: 4
PROTEIN: 40
FAT: 46

BAKED SALMON WITH GREEN VEGGIES

A sheet pan arranged with lots of veggies and salmon is what's for dinner tonight! We confess we eat this right off of the pan. It's that good! *(Pictured on pages 214–15.)*

- 1 medium (124 g) yellow zucchini, trimmed and sliced
- 1 medium (90 g) fennel bulb, trimmed and sliced
- ½ cup (100 g) diced tomatoes
- 4 cups (120 g) baby spinach
- 1 pound (454 g) wild-caught skin-on salmon fillets
- 4 tablespoons (60 g) butter, cut into small pieces
- 2 garlic cloves, minced
- 1 teaspoon (5 g) sea salt
- ½ teaspoon (1 g) black pepper
- 2 teaspoons (10 g) dried thyme
- ¼ cup (60 mL) extra-virgin olive oil

  Fennel fronds, for garnish

INSTRUCTIONS:

Preheat the oven to 400°F (200°C). Line a rimmed baking sheet with parchment paper.

Spread out the zucchini, fennel, tomatoes, and baby spinach on the prepared baking sheet. Place the salmon fillets on top of the veggies, then scatter the pieces of butter over all. Sprinkle with the garlic, sea salt, black pepper, and thyme.

Bake until the salmon is cooked to your liking and the veggies have softened, about 15 minutes. Serve with a drizzle of olive oil and a sprinkle of fennel fronds.

SERVES 4
PREP TIME: 10 MINUTES
COOKING TIME: 15 MINUTES

CALORIES: 385
CARBS: 4
PROTEIN: 24
FAT: 30

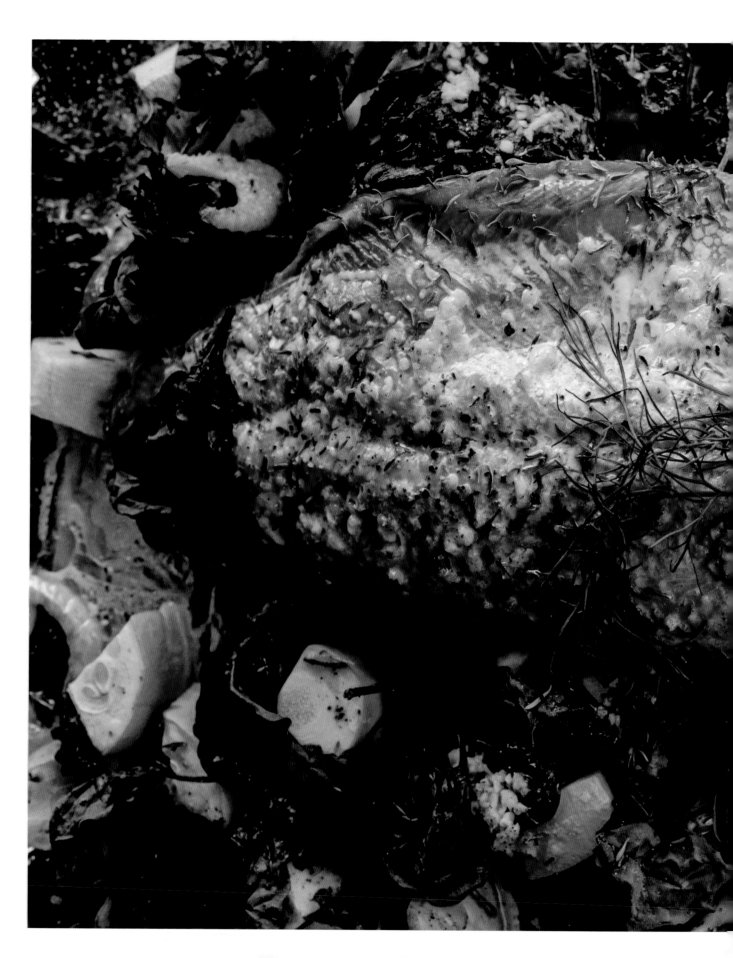

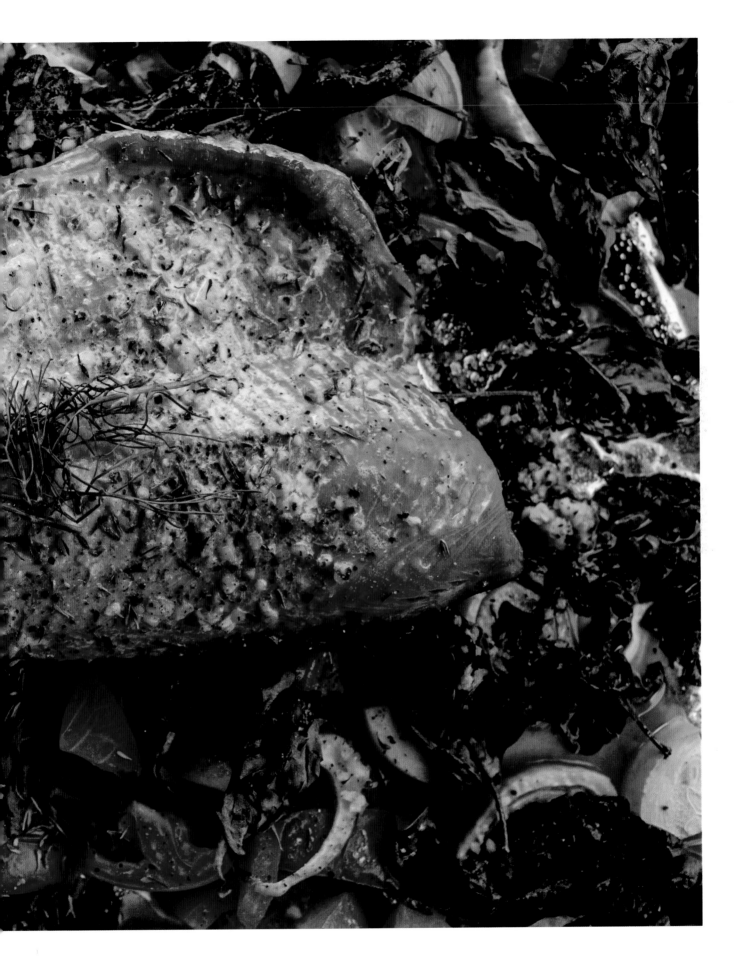

LEMON BUTTER FISH

Browning the butter in this dish takes only a few minutes but offers delicious flavor, so don't skip this step! Serve this fish as is or with a side of steamed, sautéed, or roasted veggies.

SAUCE:

- 4 tablespoons (60 g) butter
- 1 tablespoon (15 mL) fresh lemon juice
- 2 garlic cloves, minced
- 1 teaspoon (5 g) sea salt
- ½ teaspoon (1 g) black pepper

FISH:

- 1 tablespoon (15 g) butter
- 4 (4-ounce/114 g) white fish fillets

SPINACH:

- 8 cups fresh baby spinach
- 1 teaspoon (5 g) sea salt
- 2 tablespoons (30 g) butter or extra-virgin olive oil
- 1 tablespoon (15 mL) fresh lemon juice

GARNISH:

- Minced fresh parsley
- ¼ cup (31 g) roasted pistachios, chopped

INSTRUCTIONS:

Melt the butter in a small saucepan over medium heat. Stir often and allow the butter to turn golden brown. When it has a nutty fragrance, pour the brown butter into a small bowl or glass measuring cup. Add the lemon juice, garlic, sea salt, and black pepper to the butter and whisk well. Set aside.

To make the fish, melt the butter in a skillet over medium-high heat. When the butter is sizzling, add the fish fillets (skin-side up, if there is skin) and sear just until cooked through, about 1½ minutes per side (or longer for thicker fillets). Transfer the fish to a plate.

Add the spinach to the same skillet, season with the sea salt, butter, and fresh lemon juice, and sauté until wilted, about 3 minutes.

Transfer the spinach to serving plates and top with the fish. Drizzle the brown butter sauce over each plate, garnish with fresh parsley and pistachios, and serve.

SERVES 4
PREP TIME: 5 MINUTES
COOKING TIME: 10 MINUTES

CALORIES: 413
CARBS: 5
PROTEIN: 31
FAT: 30

SEAFOOD AND CAULIFLOWER RISOTTO

This "risotto" is grain-free because it uses riced cauliflower! Packed with healthy fats and protein, this dish will surely become one of your favorites. Serve as is, over a bed of greens, or alongside sautéed veggies drizzled with olive oil.

- 4 tablespoons (60 g) butter, divided
- 1 (6-ounce/170 g) salmon fillet, cut into bite-size pieces
- 4 ounces (114 g) shrimp, peeled, deveined, and cut into bite-size pieces
- 1 teaspoon (5 g) sea salt
- ½ teaspoon (1 g) black pepper
- 4 cups (1000 g) riced cauliflower
- 10 cherry tomatoes, halved
- 1 scallion, minced
- ½ cup (120 mL) canned coconut cream
- 2 garlic cloves, minced

  Minced fresh cilantro, for garnish

INSTRUCTIONS:

Melt 2 tablespoons of the butter in a large skillet over medium-high heat. Add the salmon and shrimp and sauté just until cooked through, 2–3 minutes. Season with the sea salt and black pepper. Transfer the salmon and shrimp to a plate and set aside.

Add the remaining 2 tablespoons butter to the same skillet. When the butter has melted, add the riced cauliflower, cherry tomatoes, and scallion and sauté until the vegetables are soft and slightly browned, 6–8 minutes. Lower the heat to medium-low and add the coconut cream. Simmer for 5 minutes, stirring often.

Return the salmon and shrimp to the skillet and add the garlic. Simmer for an additional 1–2 minutes, stirring frequently. Garnish with the cilantro and serve.

SERVES 4
PREP TIME: 10 MINUTES
COOKING TIME: 20 MINUTES

CALORIES: 498
CARBS: 12
PROTEIN: 16
FAT: 22

SALMON CURRY

Our salmon curry is creamy and delicious, perfect to serve alone or over a bowl of riced cauliflower. This dish freezes well, so be sure to make a big batch so that you can save its leftovers for another day!

2 tablespoons (30 g) butter

1 medium (150 g) yellow onion, diced

3 garlic cloves, minced

1 cup (100 g) cremini mushrooms, sliced

1 (14-ounce/400 mL) can coconut cream

2 cups (480 mL) chicken stock

1 pound (454 g) wild-caught salmon fillets, cut into bite-size pieces

2 teaspoons (10 g) sea salt

1 tablespoon (15 g) curry powder

1 medium (150 g) avocado, peeled, pitted, and diced

Fresh basil leaves, for garnish

INSTRUCTIONS:

Melt the butter in a large pot over medium heat. Add the onion and garlic and cook until translucent, about 5 minutes. Add the mushrooms and sauté for a few minutes more. Add the canned coconut cream and chicken stock and bring to a boil. Add the salmon, sea salt, and curry powder and bring to a simmer. Cook until the salmon is cooked through, 3–5 minutes. Stir in the diced avocado. Garnish with the basil and serve.

SERVES 4

PREP TIME: 10 MINUTES

COOKING TIME: 15 MINUTES

CALORIES: 420

CARBS: 7

PROTEIN: 33

FAT: 32

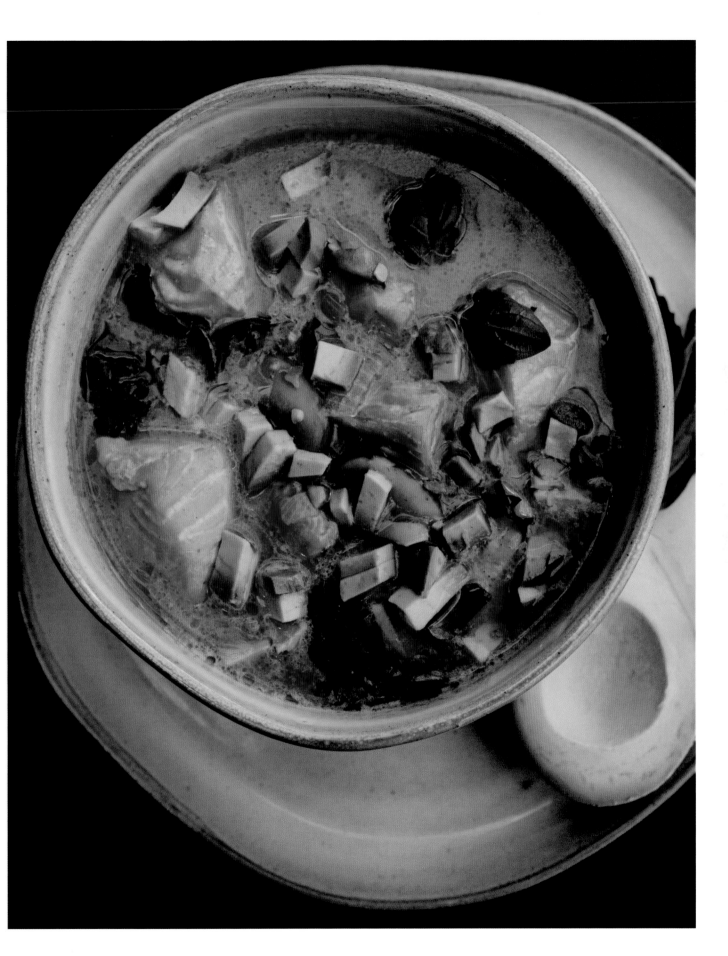

SALMON WITH CREAMY DILL SAUCE

Fresh salmon with a batch of creamy dill sauce is a sure way to get your healthy fats, leaving you feeling satisfied but never too full. We use dried dill, but if you have fresh, mince it up and enjoy!

SALMON:

- **4 (4-ounce/114 g) wild-caught, skin-on salmon fillets**
- **¼ cup (60 mL) extra-virgin olive oil**
- **2 teaspoons (10 g) sea salt**
- **1 teaspoon (2 g) black pepper**
- **4 lemon slices**

CREAMY DILL SAUCE:

- **¼ cup (60 g) full-fat sour cream**
- **¼ cup (60 g) mayonnaise**
- **1 tablespoon (15 mL) fresh lemon juice**
- **1 teaspoon (5 g) dried dill**
- **½ teaspoon (0.7 g) garlic powder**
- **½ teaspoon (2.5 g) sea salt**

GARNISH:

- **1 medium (150 g) avocado, peeled, pitted, and diced**

INSTRUCTIONS:

Preheat the oven to 350°F (180°C). Line a rimmed baking sheet with parchment paper.

Place the salmon skin side down on the prepared baking sheet. Drizzle each fillet with olive oil and sprinkle with the sea salt and black pepper. Top each with a lemon slice. Bake until the salmon begins to flake, about 20 minutes.

While the salmon is baking, combine all the creamy dill sauce ingredients in a small bowl and stir until smooth.

Serve the salmon with the creamy dill sauce and diced avocado.

SERVES 4
PREP TIME: 10 MINUTES
COOKING TIME: 20 MINUTES

CALORIES: 537
CARBS: 2
PROTEIN: 24
FAT: 48

CAESAR SALMON WITH ROASTED VEGGIES

Make this recipe your go-to when you have only a little time but want a big punch of flavor in every bite of protein and healthy fats. Aim to use the highest-quality Caesar dressing that you can, without added sugars or inflammatory oils.

- 4 (5-ounce/142 g) wild-caught, skin-on salmon fillets
- 2 cups (300 g) cherry tomatoes
- 1 cup (100 g) sliced cremini mushrooms
- 1 (14-ounce/400 g) can quartered artichoke hearts, packed in water, drained
- 1 medium (150 g) red bell pepper, seeded and sliced
- 2 garlic cloves, minced
- 2 teaspoons (10 g) sea salt
- 1 teaspoon (2 g) black pepper
- 1 teaspoon (5 g) dried thyme
- 1 teaspoon (5 g) red pepper flakes
- 1 lemon, cut into 4 wedges
- ¼ cup (60 mL) bottled Caesar dressing
- ¼ cup (60 mL) extra-virgin olive oil
- 4 tablespoons (60 mL) butter, melted
- Minced fresh parsley, for garnish

INSTRUCTIONS:

Preheat the oven to 425°F (220°C). Line a rimmed baking sheet with parchment paper. Place the salmon fillets skin side down on the prepared baking sheet.

In a large bowl, combine the cherry tomatoes, mushrooms, artichoke hearts, and red bell pepper. Add all the remaining ingredients except the parsley garnish and toss to coat. Spread out the veggie mixture on the baking sheet with the salmon. Roast until the fish just begins to flake easily with a fork and the vegetables are tender, 12–15 minutes. Garnish with the parsley and serve.

SERVES 4
PREP TIME: 10 MINUTES
COOKING TIME: 15 MINUTES

CALORIES: 584
CARBS: 11
PROTEIN: 29
FAT: 46

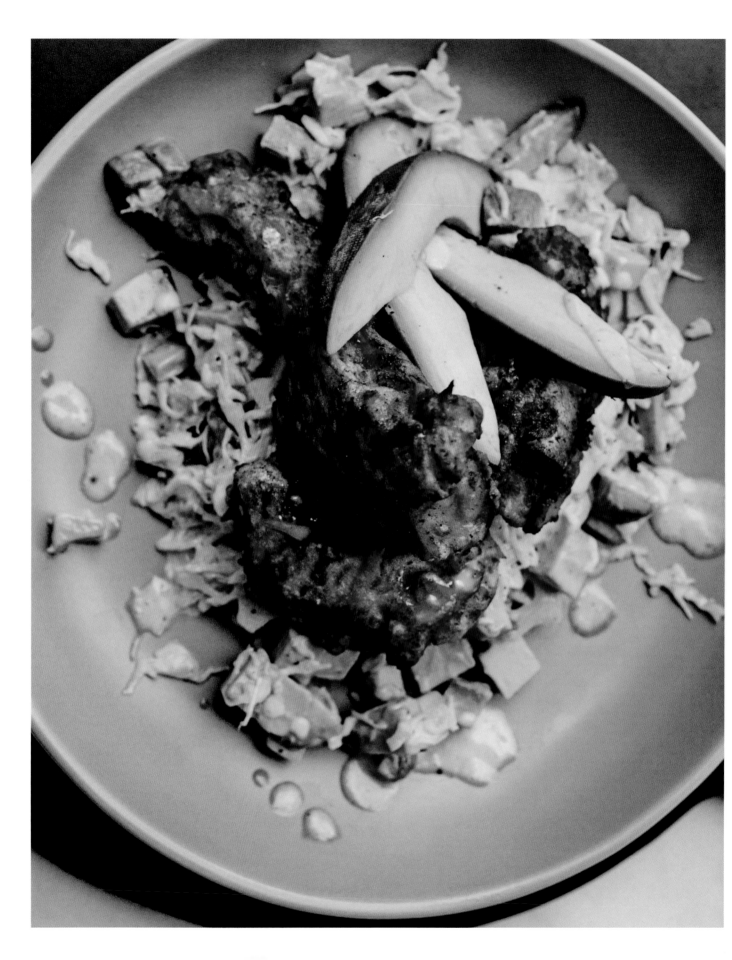

FISH TACO SALAD

We're fryin' up our own fish for a tasty keto fish taco salad! You can use any white fish you like, such as cod, rockfish, or halibut.

BATTER:

- ½ cup (50 g) almond flour
- 2 tablespoons (12 g) grated Parmesan cheese
- 1 teaspoon (5 g) sea salt
- ½ teaspoon (1 g) black pepper
- 1 teaspoon (5 g) red pepper flakes
- 1 large egg
- ⅓ cup (80 mL) water

FISH:

- 32 ounces (912 g) white fish fillets
- 1 teaspoon (5 g) sea salt
- ½ teaspoon (1 g) black pepper
- 4 tablespoons (60 g) butter

SALAD:

- ½ cup (120 g) mayonnaise
- 1 tablespoon (15 ml) fresh lime juice
- 2 teaspoons (10 mL) sriracha
- ½ teaspoon (2.5 g) sea salt
- ¼ teaspoon (0.5 g) black pepper
- 4 cups (340 g) shredded green cabbage
- 1 medium (150 g) avocado, peeled, pitted, and sliced, for garnish

INSTRUCTIONS:

Whisk together all the batter ingredients in a shallow bowl.

Pat the fish fillets dry with a paper towel. Cut the fillets into about 2 × 1-inch pieces and sprinkle with the sea salt and black pepper on both sides. Dip each piece of fish in the batter to fully coat; set aside on a plate.

Melt the butter in a cast-iron skillet over medium heat. Carefully add the battered fish in a single layer and cook until golden brown, 1–3 minutes per side. Transfer the fish to a plate.

Toss together all the salad ingredients until well combined. Serve the fried fish on top and garnish with avocado slices.

SERVES 4
PREP TIME: 15 MINUTES
COOKING TIME: 10 MINUTES

CALORIES: 543
CARBS: 9
PROTEIN: 18
FAT: 51

SHRIMP WITH PICO DE GALLO SALAD

This meal is extra quick to prepare if you use store-bought pico de gallo and precooked shrimp. Enjoy this as is, or alongside some steamed veggies drizzled with olive oil and fresh lemon juice.

VINAIGRETTE:

- ¼ cup (60 mL) extra-virgin olive oil
- 1 tablespoon (15 mL) fresh lime juice
- ¼ teaspoon (1.25 mL) hot sauce
- 1 teaspoon (5 g) sea salt
- ½ teaspoon (1 g) black pepper
- 1 teaspoon (5 g) ground cumin

SALAD:

- 2 medium (150 g) avocados, peeled, pitted, and diced
- 1 pound (454 g) cooked shrimp, peeled and deveined
- 1 cup (262 g) pico de gallo
- Handful fresh cilantro leaves, minced

GARNISH:

- Fresh lime wedges
- Fresh parsley

INSTRUCTIONS:

Whisk together all the vinaigrette ingredients in a large bowl until well combined. Gently fold in all the salad ingredients. Divide the salad among 4 serving dishes, garnish with lime wedges and parsley, and serve.

SERVES 4

PREP TIME: 10 MINUTES

CALORIES: 729

CARBS: 6

PROTEIN: 58

FAT: 51

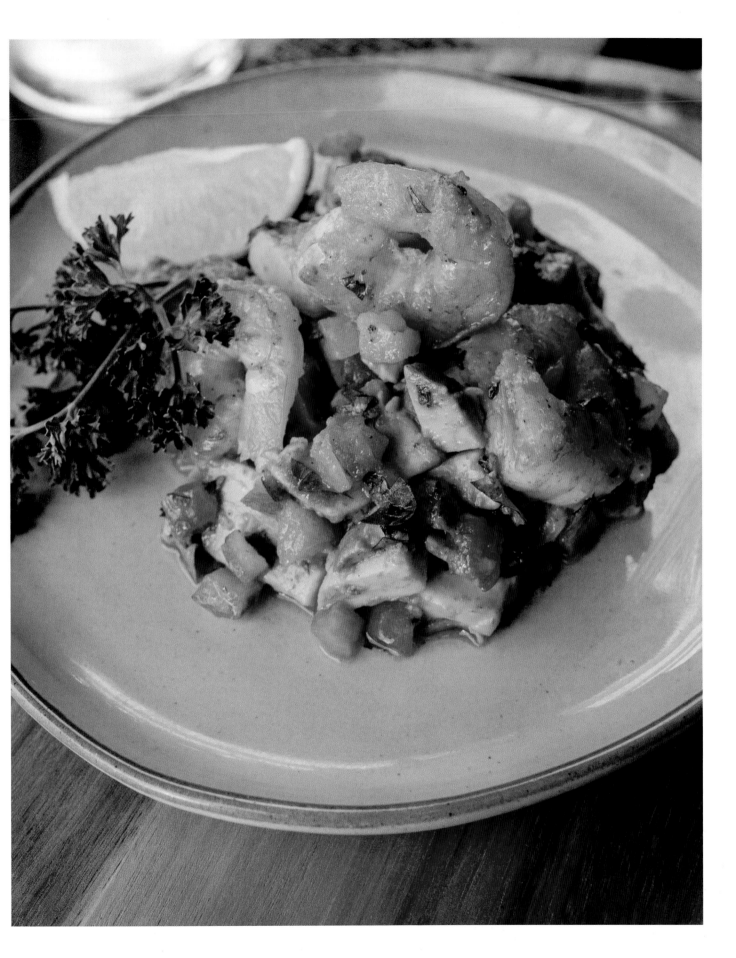

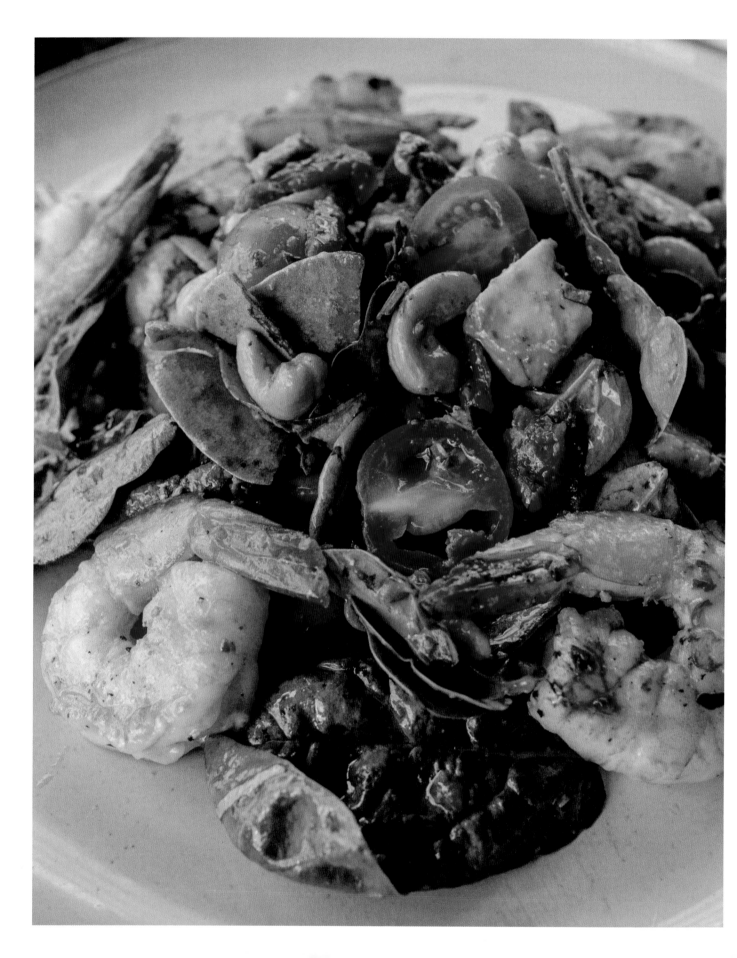

SHRIMP AND AVOCADO SALAD

This shrimp and avocado salad is packed full of healthy fats and lean protein to keep you feeling satisfied before your next meal. If you don't have cashews, try pine nuts, walnuts, macadamia nuts, or almonds, and if you don't have baby spinach, baby kale or chopped romaine works nicely!

- 2 **tablespoons (30 mL) extra-virgin olive oil**
- 1 **tablespoon (15 mL) fresh lime juice**
- ½ **teaspoon (2.5 g) sea salt**
- ¼ **teaspoon (0.5 g) black pepper**
- 5 **cilantro sprigs, minced**
- 1 **cup (150 g) cherry tomatoes, halved**
- 1 **medium (150 g) avocado, peeled, pitted, and diced**
- ¼ **cup (28 g) raw or dry-roasted cashews**
- ¼ **cup (60 g) sun-dried tomatoes, packed in olive oil, chopped**
- 2 **cups (60 g) baby spinach**
- 1 **tablespoon (15 g) ghee or butter**
- 4 **ounces (114 g) shrimp, peeled and deveined and tails left on**

INSTRUCTIONS:

In a large bowl, whisk together the olive oil, lime juice, sea salt, and black pepper. Add the cilantro, cherry tomatoes, avocado, cashews, and sun-dried tomatoes and toss until everything is coated in olive oil. Add the baby spinach and toss again to combine.

Melt the ghee in a skillet over medium-high heat. Add the shrimp and sear for 1 minute without moving them. Flip the shrimp and sear the other side for 1 minute.

Divide the salad between 2 plates and top each with half of the shrimp.

SERVES 2
PREP TIME: 10 MINUTES
COOKING TIME: 5 MINUTES

CALORIES: 506
CARBS: 16
PROTEIN: 23
FAT: 38

VEGGIE-ISH ENTREES

CHAPTER 11

I come in peace to spread love and good cheer to all healthy eating enthusiasts across the planet! While choosing to adhere to a vegan or vegetarian eating strategy is a high-risk endeavor because you will be avoiding the most nutrient-dense foods on the planet, you can certainly enjoy many meatless dishes as meals or sides.

FRIED CAULIFLOWER RICE BOWL

Here is a simple one-skillet meal combining fresh veggies, eggs, and umami coconut aminos. Avocado and an extra drizzle of oil added at the end increase this meal's fat content, so don't skimp!

- **2 tablespoons (30 mL) extra-virgin olive oil or avocado oil, divided**
- **2 cups (200 g) riced cauliflower**
- **1 teaspoon (5 g) sea salt**
- **½ teaspoon (1 g) black pepper**
- **1 cup (70 g) coleslaw mix or shredded cabbage**
- **1 tablespoon (15 mL) coconut aminos**
- **2 large eggs**
- **1 scallion, minced**
- **1 medium (150 g) avocado, peeled, pitted, and sliced**
- **1 teaspoon (3 g) sesame seeds**

INSTRUCTIONS:

Heat 1 tablespoon of the oil in a large skillet over medium-low heat. Add the riced cauliflower, sea salt, and black pepper and sauté until the riced cauliflower has begun to soften, about 3 minutes. Add the coleslaw and sauté until soft, about 3 minutes. Stir in the coconut aminos.

Crack the eggs right into the veggie mix and quickly scramble with the veggies. Top with the scallion, avocado, sesame seeds, and remaining 1 tablespoon oil and serve.

SERVES 1
PREP TIME: 5 MINUTES
COOKING TIME: 10 MINUTES

CALORIES: 747
CARBS: 12
PROTEIN: 22
FAT: 62

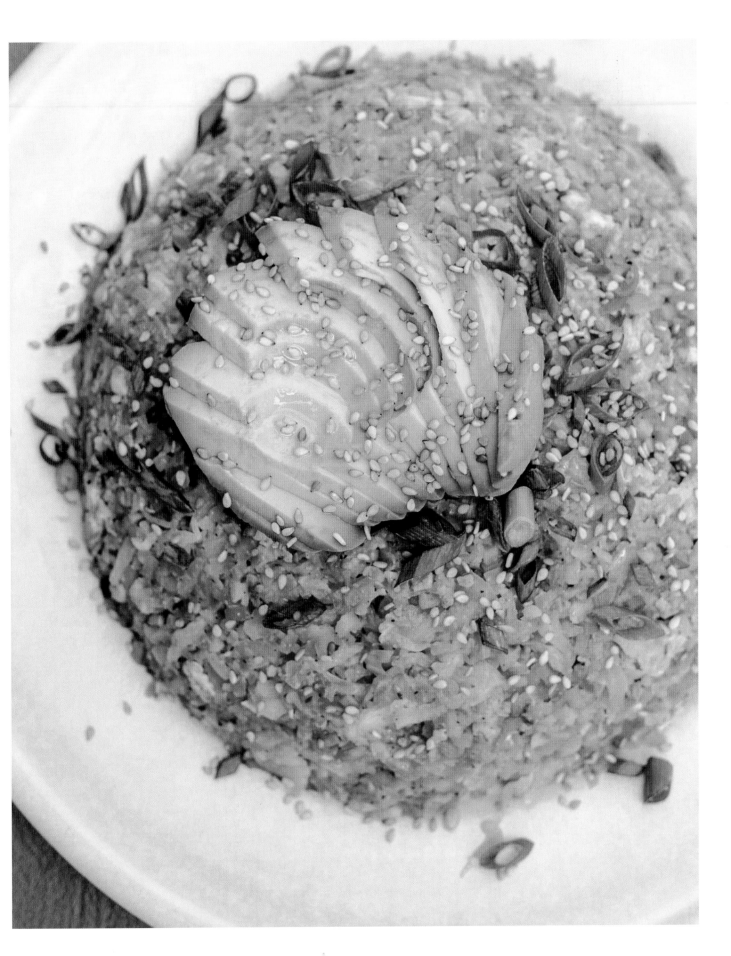

AVOCADO CAPRESE SALAD

Make this to serve alongside grilled steak, chicken, or fish and enjoy the wonderful flavors of summer. You can add a handful of pine nuts for added crunch.

- 6 tablespoons (90 g) extra-virgin olive oil
- 1 tablespoon (15 mL) fresh lemon juice
- 1 teaspoon (5 g) sea salt
- ½ teaspoon (1 g) black pepper
- 1 garlic clove, minced
- 1 cup (20 g) fresh basil leaves, chopped
- 2 cups (300 g) cherry tomatoes, halved
- 2 medium (300 g) avocados, peeled, pitted, and diced
- 4 ounces (114 g) mozzarella cheese balls, diced

INSTRUCTIONS:

In a large bowl, whisk together the oil, lemon juice, sea salt, black pepper, and garlic. Add the basil, tomatoes, avocados, and mozzarella cheese and gently toss until everything is coated and well combined. Store leftovers in an airtight container in the fridge for up to 3 days.

SERVES 4
PREP TIME: 15 MINUTES

CALORIES: 420
CARBS: 5
PROTEIN: 10
FAT: 39

CHEESY CAULIFLOWER SOUP

A batch of this cheesy cauliflower soup will nourish your body with healthy fats. You can serve this as is, or with crumbled bacon for meat lovers, all atop a big batch of riced cauliflower.

- 2 tablespoons (30 g) butter
- 1 medium (150 g) yellow onion, chopped
- 2 garlic cloves, minced
- 1 teaspoon (5 g) sea salt
- ½ teaspoon (1 g) black pepper
- 1 teaspoon (5 g) red pepper flakes

  Pinch ground nutmeg

- 4 cups (400 g) cauliflower florets
- 2 cups (480 mL) vegetable broth
- 1 cup (240 mL) heavy cream

GARNISH:

- ¼ cup (60 g) full-fat sour cream
- 1 cup (114 g) shredded Cheddar cheese
- ½ cup (32 g) minced fresh parsley
- 1 scallion, minced

  Black pepper

INSTRUCTIONS:

Melt the butter in a soup pot over medium-low heat. Add the onion and garlic and sauté until soft, about 5 minutes. Season with the sea salt, black pepper, red pepper flakes, and nutmeg. Add the cauliflower, reduce the heat to low, and stir in the vegetable broth and cream. Simmer, stirring often, for 15 minutes.

Transfer the soup to a blender. Blend on high until creamy. (When blending hot liquids, be sure to remove the cap from the center of the blender lid and hold a towel over the hole to allow steam to escape.)

Serve topped with sour cream, shredded cheese, fresh parsley, minced scallion, and a sprinkle of black pepper. Store leftovers in an airtight container in the fridge for up to 7 days.

SERVES 4
PREP TIME: 10 MINUTES
COOKING TIME: 20 MINUTES

CALORIES: 451
CARBS: 7
PROTEIN: 13
FAT: 41

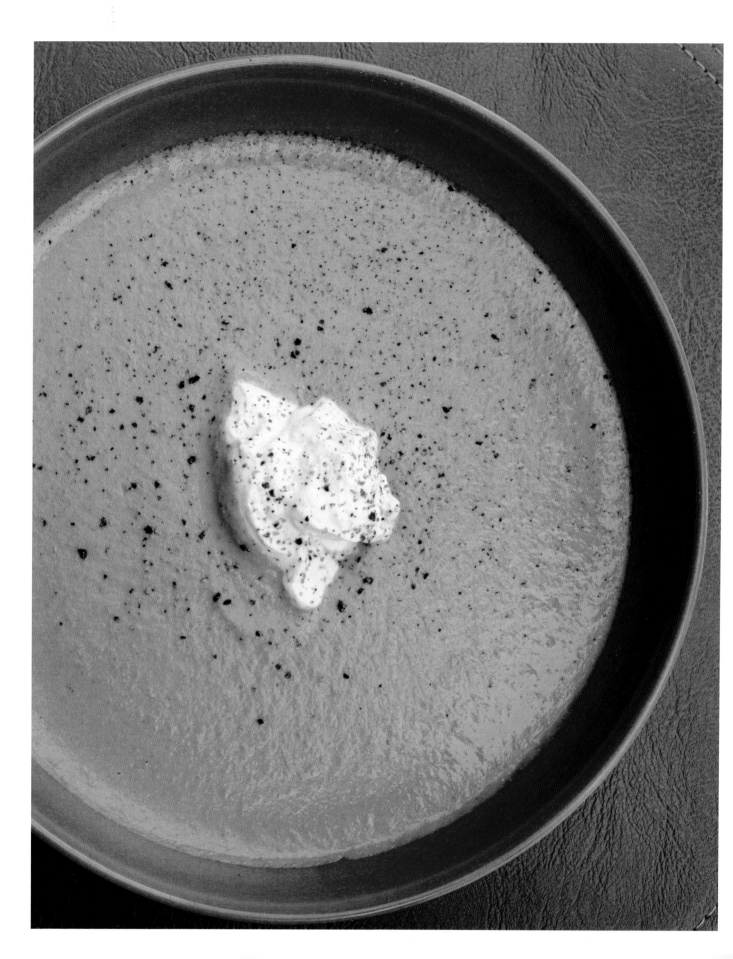

CREAM OF BUTTERNUT SOUP

Sautéing fresh sage leaves and chopped walnuts gives this creamy butternut squash soup extra warmth. Garnishing with full-fat sour cream will complete this nourishing soup by adding even more satisfying fat and texture.

- 2 **tablespoons (30 g) butter**
- 1 **medium (150 g) yellow onion, chopped**
- 2 **garlic cloves, minced**
- 1 **teaspoon (5 g) sea salt**
- ½ **teaspoon (1 g) black pepper, plus more for garnish**

  Pinch ground nutmeg
- 5 **fresh sage leaves, minced**
- ½ **cup (56 g) chopped walnuts**
- 4 **cups (560 g) cubed butternut squash**
- 2 **cups (480 mL) vegetable broth**
- 1 **cup (240 mL) heavy cream**
- ¼ **cup (60 g) full-fat sour cream, for garnish**

INSTRUCTIONS:

Melt the butter in a soup pot over medium-low heat. Add the onion and garlic and sauté until soft, about 5 minutes. Season with the sea salt, black pepper, and nutmeg. Add the sage and walnuts and sauté for 3 minutes. Add the butternut squash, reduce the heat to low, and stir in the vegetable broth and cream. Simmer, stirring often, for 15 minutes.

Transfer the soup to a blender. Blend on high until creamy. (When blending hot liquids, be sure to remove the cap from the center of the blender lid and hold a towel over the hole to allow steam to escape.)

Serve topped with a dollop of sour cream and a sprinkle of black pepper. Store leftovers in an airtight container in the fridge for up to 7 days.

SERVES 4
PREP TIME: 10 MINUTES
COOKING TIME: 25 MINUTES

CALORIES: 434
CARBS: 21
PROTEIN: 6
FAT: 37

SLOW COOKER COCONUT BUTTERNUT STEW

This dish will warm you up and leave you feeling nourished. We didn't add meat to this recipe, but you can add a pound of diced cooked chicken to increase its protein. This is wonderful served alone or over riced cauliflower.

- 2 tablespoons (30 g) butter, melted
- 1 (14-ounce/400 g) can coconut cream
- 1 cup (240 mL) vegetable broth
- 1 medium (150 g) yellow onion, sliced
- 3 garlic cloves, minced
- 1 inch fresh ginger, peeled and minced
- 1 teaspoon (5 g) sea salt
- ½ teaspoon (1 g) black pepper
- 1 teaspoon (5 g) ground turmeric
- 1 tablespoon (15 g) yellow curry powder
- 4 cups (560 g) cubed butternut squash
- ¼ cup chopped fresh cilantro, for garnish

INSTRUCTIONS:

Combine the melted butter, coconut cream, vegetable broth, onion, minced garlic, ginger, sea salt, black pepper, ground turmeric, and curry powder in a slow cooker and stir well to combine. Add the butternut squash and gently toss to combine.

Cover and cook on low for 4 hours or on high for 2 hours. Serve garnished with fresh cilantro. Store leftovers in an airtight container in the fridge for up to 1 week.

SERVES 4
PREP TIME: 10 MINUTES
COOKING TIME: 2–4 HOURS

CALORIES: 504
CARBS: 25
PROTEIN: 8
FAT: 42

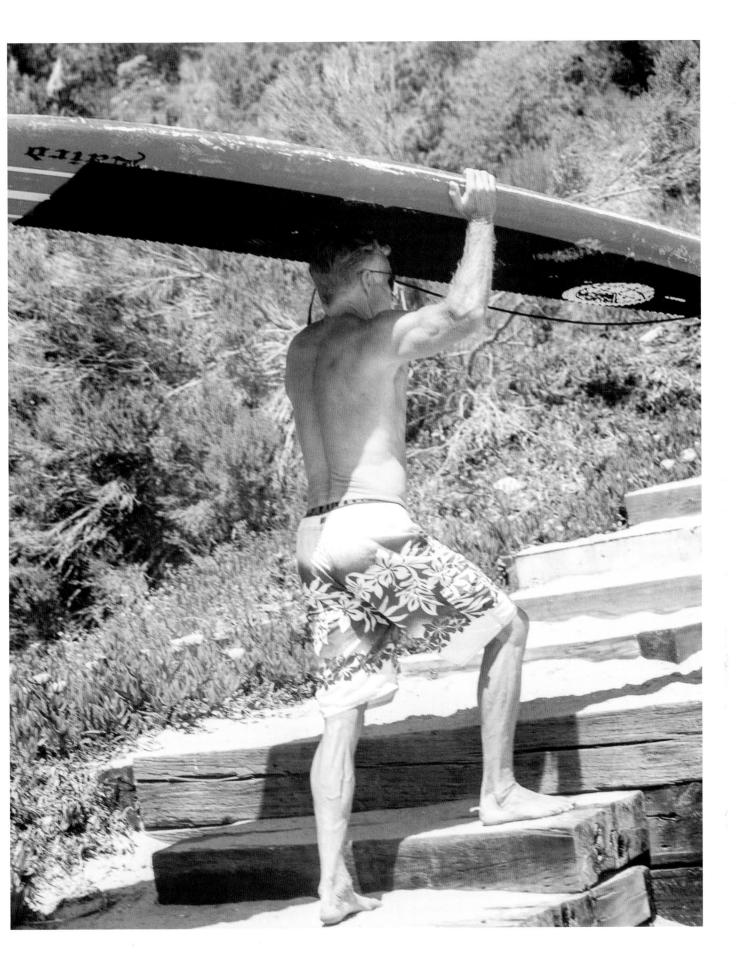

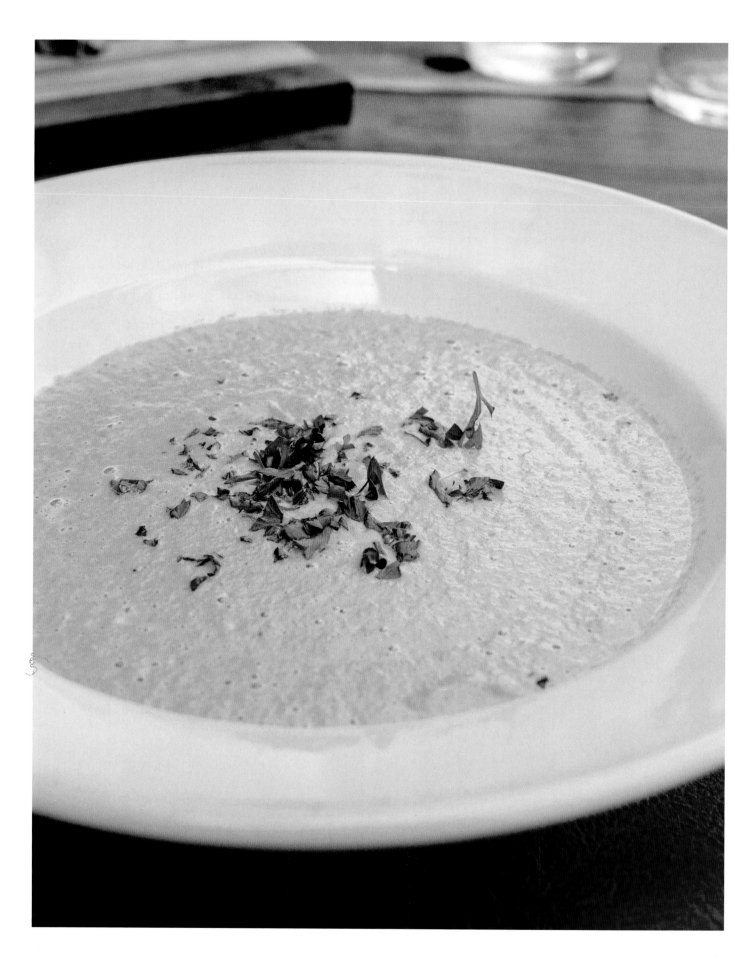

CREAM OF MUSHROOM SOUP

Creamy mushroom soup will nourish your body and your spirit on a colder day. Our version uses fresh ingredients and will ensure you receive a good dose of healthy fats. This is wonderful served with grilled steak and riced cauliflower.

- 2 **tablespoons (30 g) butter**
- 1 **medium (150 g) yellow onion, chopped**
- 2 **garlic cloves, minced**
- 1 **teaspoon (5 g) sea salt**
- ½ **teaspoon (1 g) black pepper, plus more for garnish**
- 1 **teaspoon (5 g) dried rosemary**
- 4 **cups (360 g) chopped cremini mushrooms**
- 2 **cups (480 mL) vegetable broth**
- 1 **cup (240 mL) heavy cream**
- **Minced fresh parsley, for garnish**

INSTRUCTIONS:

Melt the butter in a soup pot over medium-low heat. Add the onion and garlic and sauté until soft, about 5 minutes. Season with the sea salt, black pepper, and rosemary. Add the mushrooms and sauté until the mushrooms are soft, about 5 minutes. Reduce the heat to low and stir in the vegetable broth and cream. Simmer, stirring often, for 10 minutes.

Transfer the soup to a blender. Blend on high until creamy. (When blending hot liquids, be sure to remove the cap from the center of the blender lid and hold a towel over the hole to allow steam to escape.)

Garnish with fresh parsley and a sprinkle of black pepper and serve. Store leftovers in an airtight container in the fridge for up to 1 week.

SERVES 4
PREP TIME: 5 MINUTES
COOKING TIME: 25 MINUTES

CALORIES: 305
CARBS: 5
PROTEIN: 5
FAT: 30

STRAWBERRY KALE SALAD

Savory feta complements sweet strawberries in this salad that you can whip up in just a few minutes. We kept our version very simple, but you can jazz it up with additional greens such as broccoli sprouts or dried herbs such as basil, oregano, or tarragon.

VINAIGRETTE:

- ½ cup (120 mL) extra-virgin olive oil
- ¼ cup (60 mL) raw apple cider vinegar
- 1 teaspoon (5 g) sea salt
- ½ teaspoon (1 g) black pepper
- 1 garlic clove, minced

SALAD:

- 8 bacon strips
- 8 cups (340 g) baby kale
- 1 teaspoon (5 g) sea salt
- ½ teaspoon (1 g) black pepper
- 2 cups (400 g) strawberries, sliced
- 10 fresh mint leaves, minced
- 1 cup (150 g) crumbled feta cheese
- ½ cup (50 g) slivered almonds

INSTRUCTIONS:

Whisk together all the vinaigrette ingredients in a large bowl. Set aside.

Cook the bacon in a skillet over medium heat until crispy, 5–7 minutes. Transfer the bacon to a plate.

Add all the salad ingredients to the bowl and gently toss until everything is coated in the vinaigrette. Crumble the bacon on top and serve. Store leftovers in an airtight container in the fridge for up to 3 days.

SERVES 4
PREP TIME: 5 MINUTES
COOKING TIME: 7 MINUTES

CALORIES: 550
CARBS: 11
PROTEIN: 15
FAT: 50

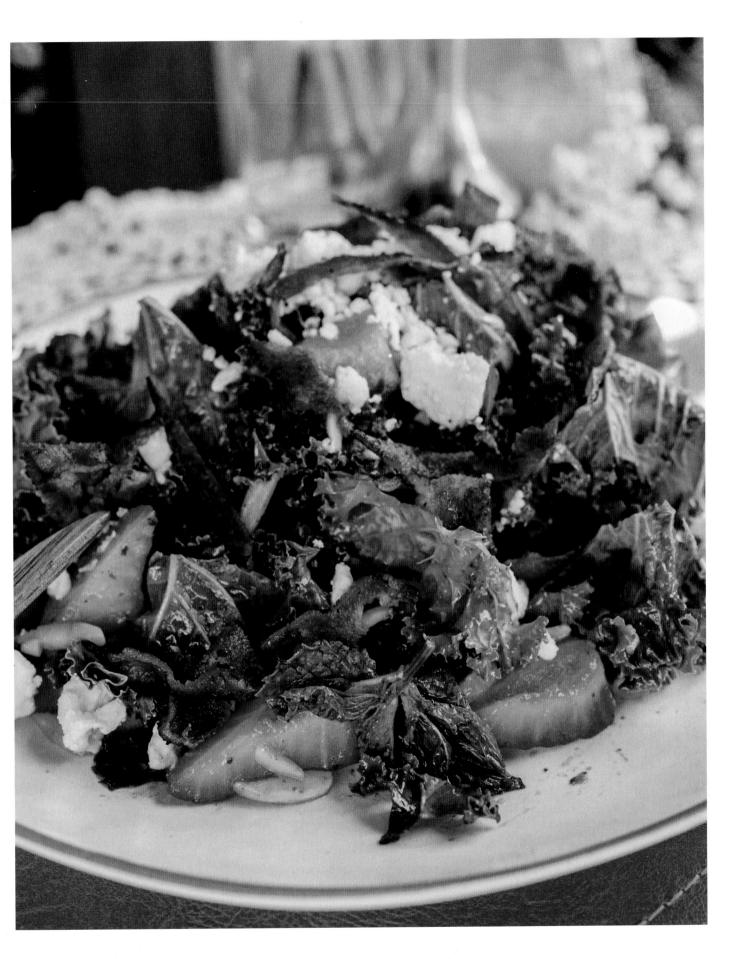

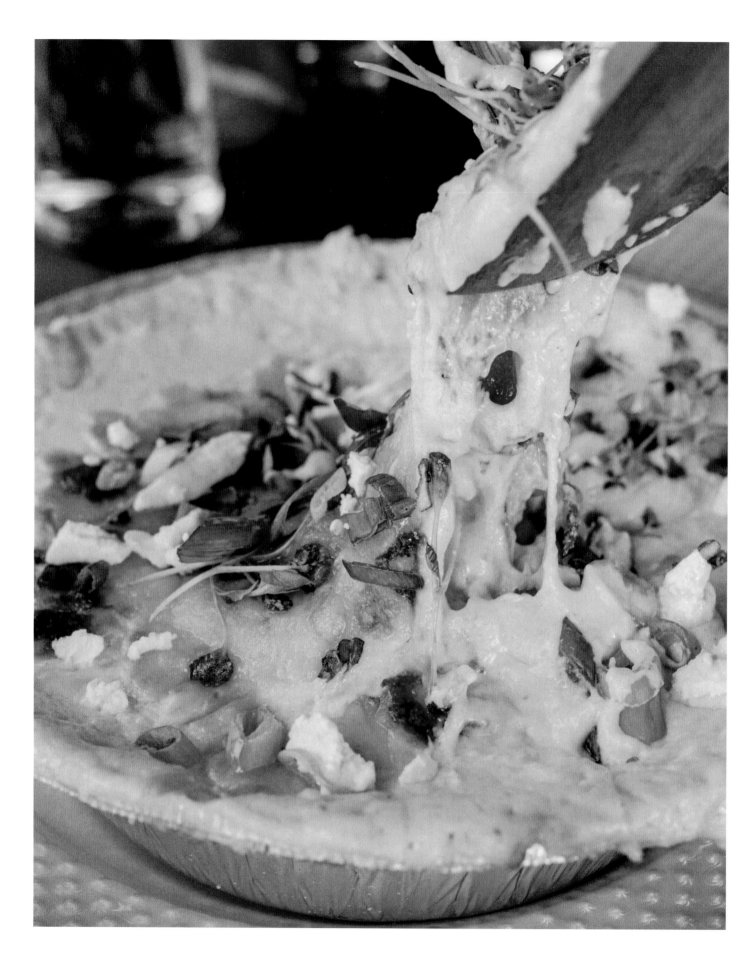

LOADED BAKED CAULIFLOWER

Creamy and ultra-comforting, this cauliflower dish hits the spot and leaves you feeling extra nourished. Cauliflower is so versatile—make sure you always have some in your fridge so you can whip up hearty dishes like this one.

- **2 bacon strips**
- **1 tablespoon (15 g) butter**
- **4 cups (400 g) cauliflower florets**
- **3 garlic cloves, minced**
- **1 teaspoon (5 g) sea salt**
- **½ teaspoon (1 g) black pepper**
- **Pinch ground nutmeg**
- **¼ cup (56 g) mascarpone cheese**
- **1 cup (240 mL) heavy cream**
- **1 cup (114 g) shredded Cheddar cheese, divided**
- **¼ cup (28 g) crumbled feta cheese, divided**
- **1 scallion, minced, divided**
- **¼ cup microgreens or broccoli sprouts, for garnish**

INSTRUCTIONS:

Preheat the oven to 400°F (200°C).

Cook the bacon in a skillet over medium heat until crispy, 5–7 minutes. Transfer the bacon to a plate, leaving the grease in the skillet, and crumble the bacon when cool.

Add the butter to the skillet and melt over medium-low heat. Add the cauliflower, bacon, and garlic, season with the sea salt, black pepper, and nutmeg, and sauté until the cauliflower is softened, about 5 minutes.

Transfer the cauliflower to a blender. Add the mascarpone cheese, cream, ½ cup of the shredded cheese, half of the feta cheese, and half of the minced scallion and blend until very creamy. Pour the mixture into a baking dish. Sprinkle with the remaining ½ cup shredded cheese.

Bake for 10 minutes, or until the cheese is bubbly. Crumble the remaining feta cheese on top, along with the remaining scallion and the microgreens, and serve. Store leftovers in an airtight container in the fridge for up to 3 days.

SERVES 4	CALORIES: 245
PREP TIME: 10 MINUTES	CARBS: 7
COOKING TIME: 20 MINUTES	PROTEIN: 12
	FAT: 20

SMOOTH-IES

The modern smoothie is presented as an antioxidant powerhouse and energizer for healthy folks, but it's typically a sugar bomb, and an anti-nutrient bomb when you throw in tons of raw leafy greens. This chapter will awaken you to new possibilities where natural, nutritious fats will be the prominent calorie source, and you can conveniently add assorted superfoods and supplements to your diet (animal organ capsules, creatine, collagen, glutamine, magnesium, whey protein) without worry about integrating everything into meal recipes.

LIVER KING SMOOTHIE

Brian "Liver King" Johnson, founder of Ancestral Supplements, is one of the most primal-living humans on the planet. Meet him at AncestralSupplements.com and you will be regaled with stories of his hard-core lifestyle featuring a Wi-Fi-free and cellular-free home illuminated with orange-hued bulbs, sleeping on the floor, daily cold exposure with extreme long dips in 38°F water, barefoot "grounding" walks after dinner, and a punishing strength training routine (including the epic "Barbarian" workout—details at the company website). Get this: He and wife, Barbara, do a five-day water fast every quarter. It's preceded not by a gourmet meal, but rather by an extreme glycogen-depleting workout Brian calls a "failed hunt." The Liver King Smoothie is often Brian's first caloric intake after a busy morning in the office and a pedal-to-the-metal midday workout.

- 2 cups (480 mL) fresh raw pastured milk from a local dairy

- 9 raw pastured egg yolks

- 4 ounces (114 g) raw grass-fed beef liver or 9 Ancestral Supplements liver capsules

- 9 Ancestral Supplements grass-fed collagen capsules

- 2–3 tablespoons (20–45 g) grass-fed, full-fat yogurt

- 1 tablespoon (15 g) organic ghee or grass-fed tallow

- 2 tablespoons (30 g) Brad's Macadamia Masterpiece nut butter or organic almond butter

- 40–50 g (1–3 scoops, depending on product) grass-fed whey protein powder

- 2 teaspoons (10 g) ancient mineral sea salt

INSTRUCTIONS:

Blend all the ingredients together until very creamy and serve immediately. Serves one extreme human athletic specimen or 2 or 3 mortal healthy, active folks.

SERVES 1 OR MORE

PREP TIME: 5 MINUTES

CALORIES: 1336

CARBS: 41

PROTEIN: 67

FAT: 97

BRAD'S SUPERFOOD RECOVERY SMOOTHIE

Honoring the baseline superfood ingredients from the Liver King Smoothie (on the facing page), this drink has extra carbs for the specific purpose of post-workout recovery. Extensive research validates the benefits of ingesting both protein and carbs soon after a high-intensity training session. There are also autophagy benefits to fasting after tough workouts, but Brad Kearns contends: "High-intensity workouts, fasting, low-carbohydrate eating, and being in the 50+ age groups are all distinct stressors to the body. When combined, it's possible to overstress the organism and delay recovery accordingly. I've experimented with all manner of pairing food, fasting, and hard workouts, and a delicious, post-workout smoothie seems to help enhance recovery and prevent the 'crash and burn' effect that can happen 12–36 hours after a challenging session."

LIVER KING BASE:

- 2 cups (480 mL) unsweetened coconut milk, almond milk, raw kefir, or raw milk
- 6 raw pastured egg yolks
- 4 ounces (114 g) raw grass-fed beef liver or 9 Ancestral Supplements liver capsules
- 9 Ancestral Supplements grass-fed collagen capsules or 1–2 medium/large scoops (20–40 g) grass-fed collagen protein
- 2–3 tablespoons (20–45 g) grass-fed, full-fat yogurt

EXTRA CARBS, PROTEIN, AND RECOVERY AGENTS:

- 1–2 big scoops (20–40 g) microfiltered whey protein isolate

  Frozen banana chunks

  Frozen mango chunks
- 5 g creatine powder
- 5 g glutamine powder
- 2 g magnesium powder
- 1 (0.21-ounce/5.93 g) packet unflavored LMNT electrolyte powder (DrinkLMNT.com)

- 6–9 Ancestral Supplements MOFO testosterone support capsules for males, or FEMM capsules for females
- 9–12 other Ancestral Supplements capsules, such as prostate, blood vitality, beef organs, and/ or beef lung

INSTRUCTIONS:

Blend all the ingredients together until very creamy (add ice chunks if necessary) and serve immediately.

SERVES 2

PREP TIME: 5 MINUTES

CALORIES: 913

CARBS: 65

PROTEIN: 80

FAT: 37

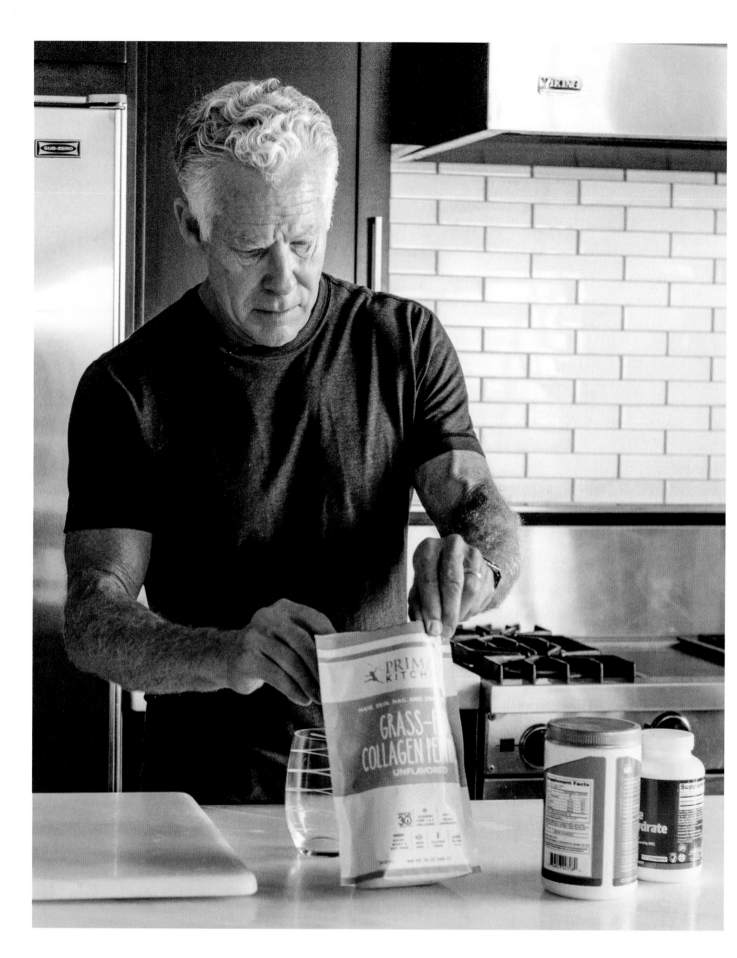

CHOCOLATE CAULIFLOWER SMOOTHIE

This creamy smoothie is packed with protein, healthy fats, and fiber. Keep frozen cauliflower in your kitchen, as it's a great thickener in smoothies and offers a boost of nutrition.

- 1 **cup (240 mL) plain unsweetened almond milk**
- 2 **large raw eggs**
- 2 **tablespoons (32 g) raw almond butter**
- 30–40 g **(1–3 scoops, depending on product) chocolate whey protein powder**
- ¼ **teaspoon (1.25 g) sea salt**
- 1 **cup (85 g) frozen riced cauliflower**
- 2 **tablespoons (20 g) unsweetened and shredded coconut**
- **Handful ice cubes**
- 1 **tablespoon cacao nibs, for garnish**

INSTRUCTIONS:

Blend all the ingredients until very creamy, garnish with the cacao nibs, and serve.

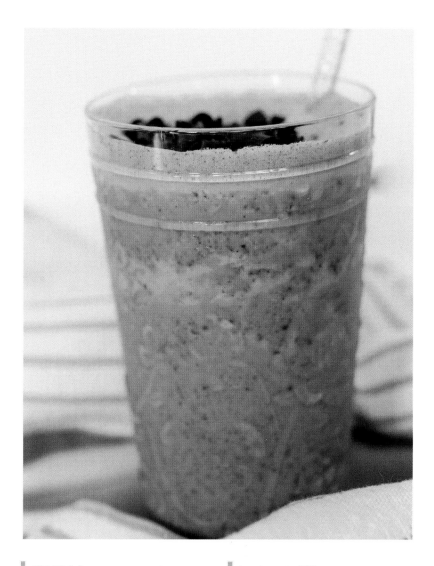

SERVES 1

PREP TIME: 5 MINUTES

CALORIES: 702

CARBS: 33

PROTEIN: 36

FAT: 50

KEY LIME SMOOTHIE

We're serving up this tropical goodness after our workouts, and it really hits the spot! To amp up the protein in this already-healthy smoothie, add some collagen peptides or vanilla whey protein powder.

- 1 **cup (240 mL) raw milk**
- 2 **large raw eggs**
- ¼ **teaspoon (1.25 g) sea salt**
- 2 **cups (60 g) baby spinach**
- 2 **tablespoons (20 g) unsweetened shredded coconut**
- 2 **tablespoons (30 mL) fresh lime juice**
- **Handful ice cubes**

INSTRUCTIONS:

Blend all the ingredients until very creamy and serve.

SERVES 1

PREP TIME: 5 MINUTES

CALORIES: 572

CARBS: 25

PROTEIN: 31

FAT: 42

PUMPKIN SPICE SMOOTHIE

The combination of heavy cream, almond butter, and pumpkin pie spice will warm your belly and leave you feeling steady and grounded. Look for canned pumpkin puree and not canned pumpkin pie filling, which has added sugars.

1 **cup (240 mL) unsweetened almond milk**

¼ **cup (60 mL) heavy cream**

2 **large raw eggs**

2 **tablespoons (32 g) raw almond butter**

¼ **teaspoon (1.25 g) sea salt**

½ **teaspoon (2.5 g) pumpkin pie spice**

½ **cup (110 g) canned pumpkin puree**

Handful ice cubes

INSTRUCTIONS:

Blend all the ingredients until very creamy and serve.

SERVES 1

PREP TIME: 5 MINUTES

CALORIES: 605

CARBS: 17

PROTEIN: 21

FAT: 54

STRAWBERRIES AND CREAM SMOOTHIE

This smoothie is made with heavy cream, making it taste extra decadent. Blended with strawberries, it's a delicious treat, so make this smoothie soon!

- 1 cup (240 mL) raw milk or unsweetened nondairy milk
- ¼ cup (60 mL) heavy cream
- 2 large raw eggs
- 30–40 g (1–3 scoops, depending on product) organic grass-fed vanilla whey protein powder
- ¼ teaspoon (1.25 g) sea salt
- ½ cup (110 g) frozen strawberries
- Handful ice cubes

INSTRUCTIONS:

Blend all the ingredients until very creamy and serve.

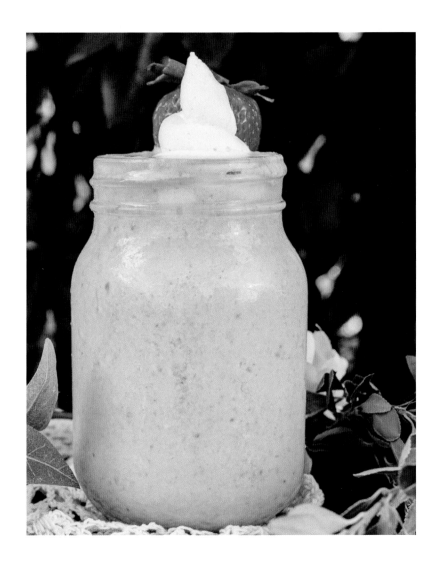

SERVES 1

PREP TIME: 5 MINUTES

CALORIES: 633

CARBS: 23

PROTEIN: 32

FAT: 47

CINNAMON RASPBERRY SMOOTHIE

The addition of collagen peptides in this smoothie boosts its protein and aids in healthy skin repair. Keep collagen in your pantry to add to smoothies on a regular basis—it's flavorless, so you can add it to anything!

- **1 cup (240 mL) raw milk or unsweetened nondairy milk**
- **2 large raw eggs**
- **30–40 g (1–3 scoops, depending on product) organic grass-fed whey protein powder**
- **20 grams (1–2 scoops, depending on product) collagen peptides**
- **¼ teaspoon (1.25 g) sea salt**
- **1 teaspoon (5 g) ground cinnamon**
- **½ cup (70 g) frozen raspberries**
- **2 tablespoons (32 g) raw almond butter**
- **Handful ice cubes**

INSTRUCTIONS:

Blend all the ingredients until very creamy and serve.

SERVES 1
PREP TIME: 5 MINUTES

CALORIES: 666
CARBS: 34
PROTEIN: 49
FAT: 40

COCONUT BERRY MINT SMOOTHIE

Fresh mint in your smoothie will wake up your taste buds and aid in digestion, so pick up a pack from your market or plant some so that you can use it in your kitchen regularly!

- 1 cup (240 mL) raw milk or unsweetened nondairy milk

- 2 large raw eggs

- 30–40 g (1–3 scoops, depending on product) organic grass-fed whey protein powder

- ¼ teaspoon (1.25 g) sea salt

- ½ cup (70 g) frozen blackberries (reserve small amount for garnish)

- 2 tablespoons (20 g) unsweetened and shredded coconut (reserve small amount for garnish)

- 5–10 fresh mint leaves (reserve small amount for garnish)

- Handful ice cubes

INSTRUCTIONS:

Blend all the ingredients until very creamy. Garnish with blackberries, coconut, and fresh mint leaves, and serve.

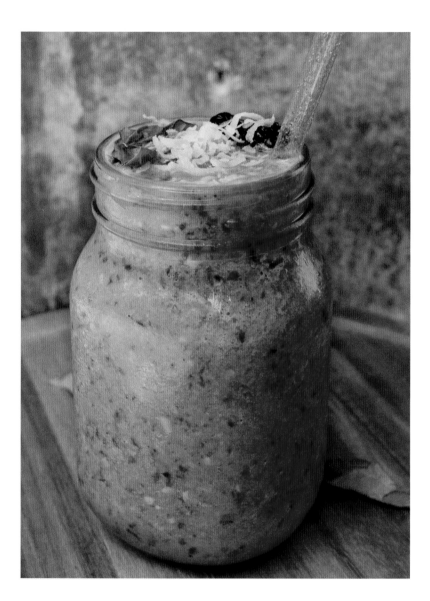

SERVES 1

PREP TIME: 5 MINUTES

CALORIES: 587

CARBS: 35

PROTEIN: 33

FAT: 36

CHOCOLATE PEANUT BUTTER SMOOTHIE

1 cup (240 mL) raw milk or unsweetened nondairy milk

2 large raw eggs

30–40 g (1–3 scoops, depending on product) organic grass-fed chocolate whey protein powder

¼ teaspoon (1.25 g) sea salt

2 tablespoons (32 g) natural peanut butter

Handful ice cubes

INSTRUCTIONS:

Blend all the ingredients until very creamy and serve.

SERVES 1
PREP TIME: 5 MINUTES

CALORIES: 595
CARBS: 23
PROTEIN: 40
FAT: 40

BIG MIXED BERRY SMOOTHIE

This smoothie will keep you full for hours and contains raw milk and raw eggs, both of which are really great choices with today's many options at your market. Use any frozen berry in this smoothie; you can often find mixed varieties in your freezer aisle.

- **1 cup (240 mL) raw milk or unsweetened nondairy milk**
- **2 large raw eggs**
- **30–40 g (1–3 scoops, depending on product) organic grass-fed whey protein powder**
- **¼ teaspoon (1.25 g) sea salt**
- **2 cups (60 g) baby spinach**
- **¾ cup (150 g) frozen mixed berries (strawberries, blueberries, raspberries, blackberries)**
- **½ medium (75 g) avocado, peeled and pitted**
- **2 tablespoons (20 g) hemp seeds**

INSTRUCTIONS:

Blend all the ingredients until very creamy and serve.

SERVES 1
PREP TIME: 5 MINUTES

CALORIES: 785
CARBS: 40
PROTEIN: 39
FAT: 48

BANANA JOINT-BOOSTER SMOOTHIE

Collagen delivers comprehensive anti-aging benefits, promoting healthy skin and connective tissue. The best dietary sources are bone broth and bone-in cuts of meat, which are often difficult to consume on a regular basis. If you have nagging joint or connective tissue issues, strive to consume 30 grams of collagen every day.

2 cups (480 mL) cold unsweetened coconut or almond milk, organic raw milk or kefir, or water

Handful ice cubes

1 frozen sliced banana

3 tablespoons (45 g) plain full-fat yogurt

30 g (1.5–3 scoops, depending on product) unflavored collagen peptides, such as Primal Collagen or Great Lakes Collagen

OPTIONAL ADD-INS:

1–2 teaspoons (5–10 mL) pure vanilla extract

1–2 teaspoons (2.5–5 g) cinnamon

1–2 tablespoons (7.5–15 g) cacao nibs

1–2 tablespoons (5–10 g) coconut flakes

Chocolate-, vanilla-, or turmeric-flavored collagen

INSTRUCTIONS:

Blend all the ingredients until very creamy and serve.

SERVES 1–3
PREP TIME: 5 MINUTES

CALORIES: 921
CARBS: 69
PROTEIN: 55
FAT: 46

BANANA NUT BUTTER ALL-DAY ENERGY SMOOTHIE

This is a great choice before a long hike or bike ride. It's calorically dense and extremely satisfying, yet easy to digest quickly.

- 2 cups (480 mL) cold unsweetened coconut or almond milk, organic raw milk or kefir, or water

- Handful ice cubes

- 1 frozen sliced banana

- 3 tablespoons (45 g) plain full-fat yogurt

- ¼ cup (60 g) almond, peanut, or other nut butter, such as Brad's Macadamia Masterpiece

- 30–40 g (1–3 scoops, depending on product) whey protein powder or collagen protein powder

INSTRUCTIONS:

Blend all the ingredients until very creamy and serve.

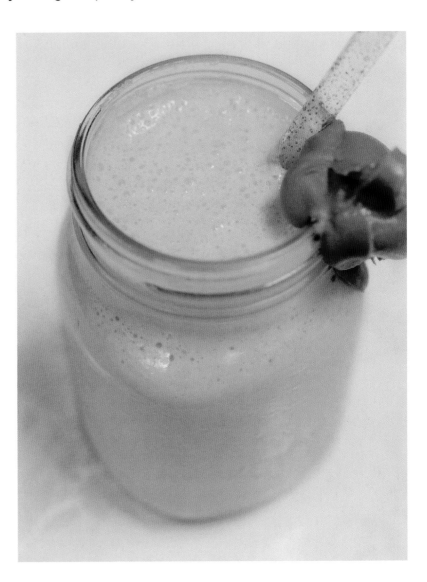

SERVES 2	CALORIES: 646
PREP TIME: 5 MINUTES	CARBS: 32
	PROTEIN: 38
	FAT: 39

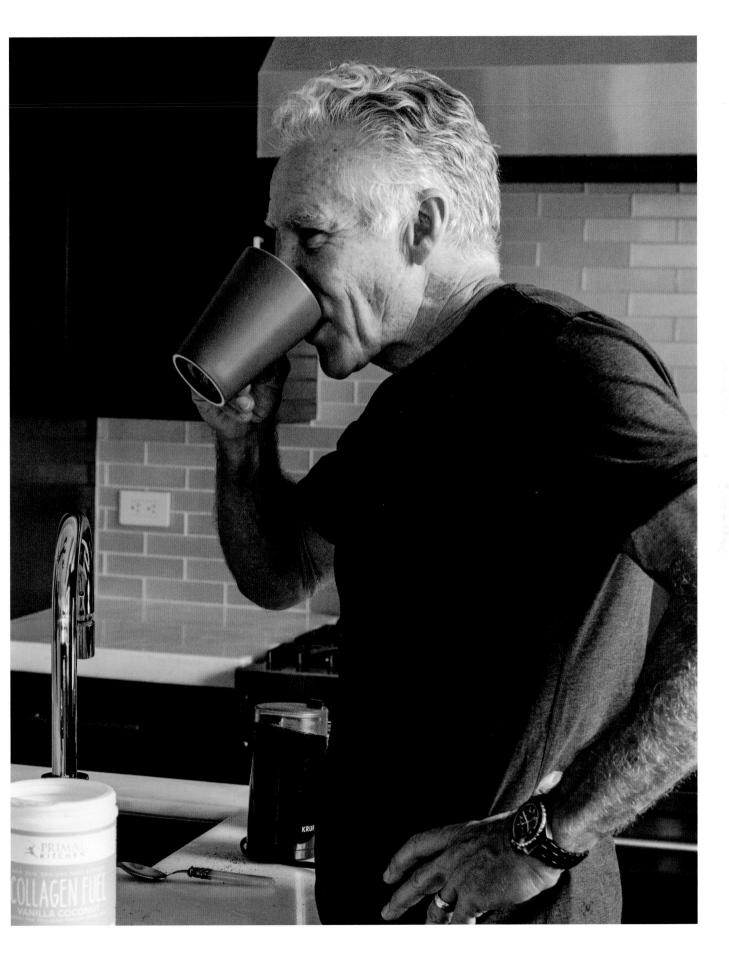

DESSERTS AND TREATS

CHAPTER 13

Granted, the Two Meals a Day program offers a strong recommendation to avoid snacking, but the desserts and treats category is in line with the "enjoy life" edict. If you are going to indulge, let's make sure you are avoiding cheap processed ingredients and can actually obtain some nutritional benefits along with sensational taste.

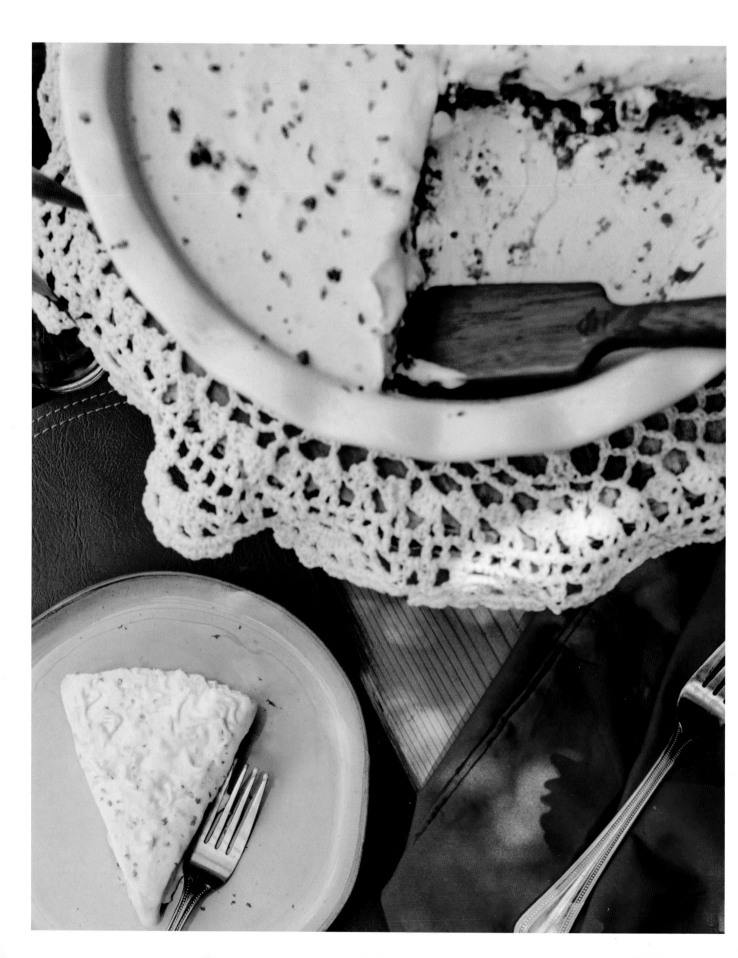

ALMOST KETO KEY LIME PIE

This zesty pie will brighten your day and give you just enough of that sweet taste without leaving you feeling antsy for more and more like some other desserts tend to do. We prefer using real ingredients in our desserts, and we know you will too.

CRUST:

- 1 **cup (125 g) pecans or walnuts, ground into a coarse flour**
- 2 **tablespoons (30 g) melted butter**
- 1 **teaspoon (5 g) honey**

FILLING:

- 1½ **cups (360 mL) heavy cream**
- 1 **tablespoon (15 g) honey**
- 5 **teaspoons grated lime zest**
- 2 **tablespoons (30 mL) fresh lime juice**
- 8 **ounces (226 g) organic cream cheese**

INSTRUCTIONS:

Preheat the oven to 350°F (180°C). Grease a pie tin.

Mix the crust ingredients together and press into the prepared pie tin. Bake for 10 minutes, then set aside to cool while you make the filling.

Whisk the cream in a medium bowl until soft peaks form, either with a hand mixer or by hand. Combine the honey and lime zest and juice in a small bowl and microwave for 10 seconds, then mix in the cream cheese. Mix the cream cheese mixture into the whipped cream, then spoon it into the pie crust. Chill in the fridge for several hours or in the freezer for 1 hour.

SERVES **8**

PREP TIME: **15 MINUTES, PLUS 1 HOUR TO FREEZE**

COOKING TIME: **10 MINUTES**

CALORIES: **336**

CARBS: **5**

PROTEIN: **3**

FAT: **35**

ALMOST KETO PUMPKIN PIE

You are going to love this fresh pumpkin pie, made with real ingredients that will leave your body feeling nourished and satisfied. This is perfect to make in the fall or during the holidays that bring us together.

CRUST:

- 1 cup (215 g) pecans, walnuts, or macadamia nuts, ground into a coarse flour
- 2 tablespoons (30 g) butter, melted, or coconut oil
- 1 teaspoon (5 g) raw honey

FILLING:

- 1 (15-ounce/425 g) can pumpkin puree
- 3 large eggs
- 2 tablespoons (30 g) honey
- 1 tablespoon (7 g) pumpkin pie spice

GARNISH:

- Whipped cream (optional)
- Fresh mint leaves

INSTRUCTIONS:

Preheat the oven to 475°F (240°C). Grease an 8-inch cast-iron skillet.

After the nuts are pulsed, add the butter and honey to the food processor and continue blending until everything is mixed. Evenly press the crust mixture into the prepared skillet. Bake for 15 minutes, then set aside to cool while you make the filling. Turn the oven down to 350°F.

In a large bowl, whisk together the filling ingredients and spoon it into the pie crust. Bake for 30 minutes.

Garnish with a dollop of whipped cream (optional) and fresh mint leaves.

SERVES 8
PREP TIME: 10 MINUTES
COOKING TIME: 40 MINUTES

CALORIES: 183
CARBS: 6
PROTEIN: 4
FAT: 15

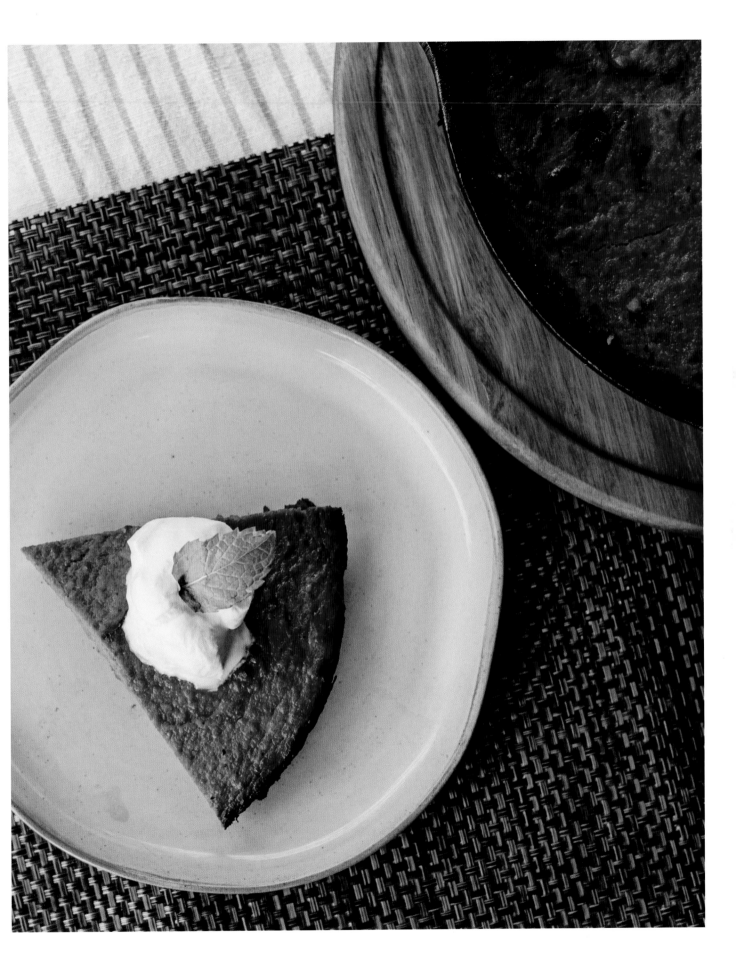

MACADAMIA VANILLA LIME COOKIES

The combination of vanilla and lime is an unexpected yet delicious flavor, so try these and invite your friends over to enjoy them too.

- 2 cups (250 g) ground macadamia nuts
- 2 large eggs
- 1 tablespoon (15 g) honey
- 1 tablespoon (15 mL) pure vanilla extract
- 1 tablespoon (15 mL) fresh lime juice

INSTRUCTIONS:

Preheat the oven to 350°F (180°C). Grease a rimmed baking sheet.

Process all the ingredients in a food processor. Drop the dough by the spoonful onto the prepared baking sheet and flatten the cookies with a fork to make silver dollar–size cookies. Bake for 10 minutes, let cool for a few minutes, and serve.

SERVES 4

PREP TIME: 10 MINUTES

COOKING TIME: 10 MINUTES

CALORIES: 151

CARBS: 5

PROTEIN: 3

FAT: 14

CHOCOLATE MOUSSE À LA BIG GEORGE

This is one of the greatest dessert recipes on the planet, but it's so healthy you can eat it for breakfast. Or for a snack after Speedgolf or a cold plunge. It's high in healthy fats and antioxidants and has almost no carbs. There are only three ingredients, so it's an easy qualifier for this book. Big George, aka Dr. Ray Sidney, perfected this recipe while getting A's at Harvard (bachelor's), MIT (PhD), and UC Berkeley (MBA). How about you? What have you been doing the past twenty years? Make this recipe so you can make something out of your life. These proportions make a good-size dose to feed your family or a few friends.

- 10 ounces (284 g) dark chocolate (80% cacao or higher)
- ½ cup (1 stick/114 g) butter or 2–3 ounces (60–85 g) cacao butter
- 6 large eggs

INSTRUCTIONS:

Pour an inch or two of water into the bottom of a double boiler and bring to a simmer over medium-low heat. Combine the chocolate and butter in the top of the double boiler and place it over the bottom pot. Melt them together, stirring frequently. (Alternatively, you can place a heatproof bowl over a saucepan of simmering water, or melt the chocolate and butter in the microwave.)

Separate the eggs into a big bowl for the whites and a smaller bowl for the yolks. Be very precise with this step, as you must have super-pristine whites for optimal whipping.

Whip the whites until they're stiff and dry. Use a hand mixer or a tabletop mixer and spend plenty of time getting the whites as voluminous as possible.

Add the yolks to the melted chocolate and butter, stirring well to combine. Fold the chocolate mixture into the egg whites, stirring gently.

Put the mixture into a glass container, cover, and refrigerate for 2 hours or freeze for 30 minutes until it turns firm.

SERVES 4

PREP TIME: 15 MINUTES, PLUS 30 MINUTES TO FREEZE

COOKING TIME: 5 MINUTES

CALORIES: 523

CARBS: 10

PROTEIN: 11

FAT: 46

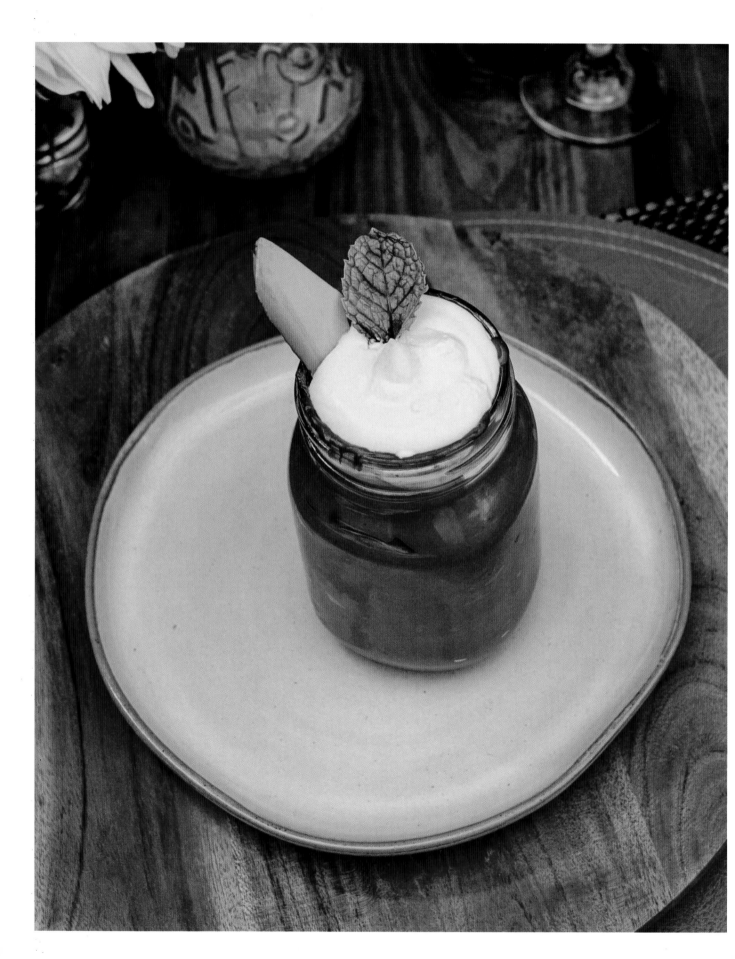

AVOCADO MOUSSE

Creamy and super simple to make, this mousse will make you want to keep avocados in your kitchen just so you can whip it up anytime you like.

- 2 ounces (57 g) dark chocolate (80% cacao or higher)

- ¼–½ cup (60–120 mL) canned full-fat coconut cream

- ½ teaspoon (2.5 mL) pure vanilla extract

- ½ teaspoon (1.25 g) ground cinnamon

- ⅛ teaspoon (0.7 g) finely ground Himalayan sea salt

- Pinch ground cayenne pepper (or more to taste)

- 1 medium (150 g) avocado, peeled and pitted

- 1 teaspoon (5 g) raw honey (optional)

- ¼ teaspoon (0.75 g) flaky salt, such as Maldon (optional)

GARNISH:

- Whipped cream (optional)

- Fresh mint leaves

INSTRUCTIONS:

Pour an inch or two of water into the bottom of a double boiler and bring to a simmer over medium-low heat. Combine the chocolate and coconut cream in the top of the double boiler and place it over the bottom pot. Melt them together, stirring frequently. (Alternatively, you can place a heatproof bowl over a saucepan of simmering water, or melt the chocolate and butter in the microwave.)

Once the chocolate is melted, stir in the vanilla, cinnamon, sea salt, and cayenne. Add the avocado and use an immersion blender (or fork) to mix until smooth. Add more coconut cream, as needed, to achieve the desired consistency. Taste and add honey if desired.

Divide the mousse between 2 ramekins. If desired, sprinkle with flaky salt. Garnish with a dollop of whipped cream (optional) and fresh mint leaves. Serve immediately or cover and refrigerate until ready to serve.

SERVES 2
PREP TIME: 10 MINUTES
COOKING TIME: 5 MINUTES

CALORIES: 395
CARBS: 24
PROTEIN: 4
FAT: 32

REALLY FAST, EASY MEALS

FOR PEOPLE WHO ARE TOO BUSY TO COOK

CHAPTER 14

This is my favorite chapter title of them all! This is also my biggest pet peeve when I look at my shelf with dozens of outstanding cookbooks full of fabulous recipes. I've enjoyed some amazing one-off preparations, but I notice that if they require too many ingredients, too many steps, and too much time, they won't make it into my regular rotation. This section is dedicated to real people leading real lives—enjoy!

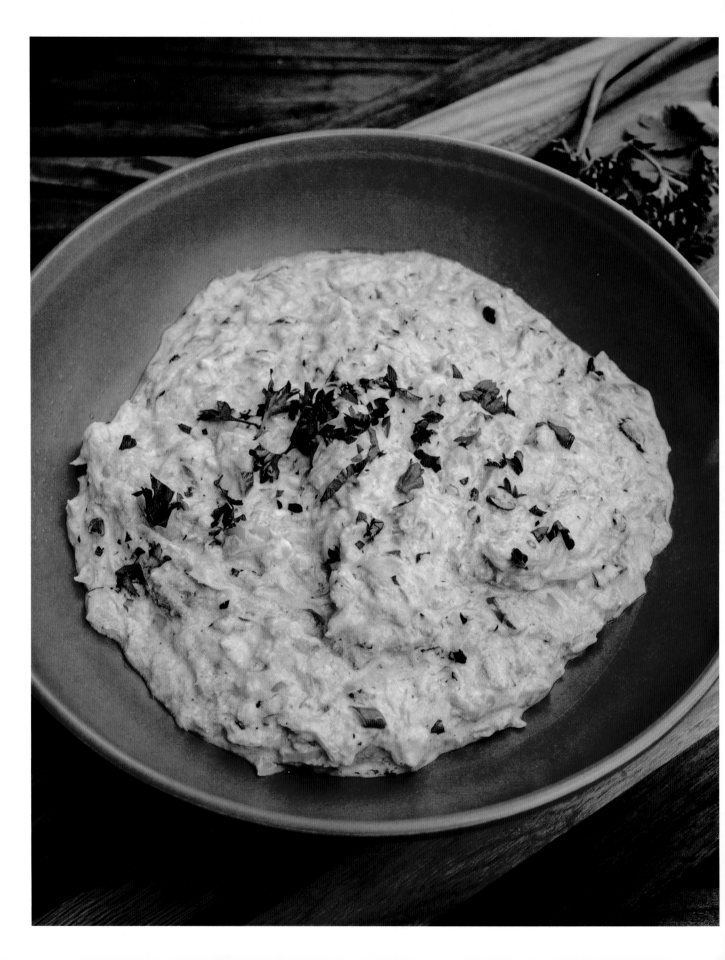

QUICK AND CREAMY TUNA SKILLET

Keep cans of tuna stocked in your pantry for times when you need some protein, fast. Add in some good, healthy fats and a low-carb veggie such as shredded cabbage and you'll have a delicious, nourishing meal in minutes.

- 2 **tablespoons (30 g) butter**
- 3 **garlic cloves, minced**
- 2 **cups (140 g) shredded green cabbage**
- 2 **teaspoons (10 g) sea salt**
- 1 **teaspoon (2 g) black pepper**
- 2 **(5-ounce/284 g) cans tuna, drained**
- 2 **cups (570 g) full-fat Greek yogurt**
- 1 **teaspoon (5 g) yellow mustard**
- **Handful fresh parsley, minced, plus more for garnish**
- 1 **scallion, minced**
- **Grated zest of ½ lemon**

INSTRUCTIONS:

Melt the butter in a skillet over medium heat. Add the garlic and shredded cabbage, season with the sea salt and black pepper, and sauté until soft and wilted, about 5 minutes. Add the tuna and stir it in with the cabbage. Turn off the heat and stir in the Greek yogurt, yellow mustard, parsley, scallion, and lemon zest until everything is well combined. Garnish with parsley and serve.

SERVES 2
PREP TIME: 5 MINUTES
COOKING TIME: 5 MINUTES

CALORIES: 475
CARBS: 16
PROTEIN: 52
FAT: 24

HAM AND CHEESE CAULIFLOWER BOWL

A quick skillet meal is perfect when you want a nourishing home-cooked meal without all the fuss of too many steps and necessary gadgets—just get it all in the skillet and stir it up! You can jazz up your bowl with extra veggies or crispy bacon.

- 2 **tablespoons (30 g) butter**
- 4 **cups (400 g) riced cauliflower**
- 2 **teaspoons (10 g) sea salt**
- 1 **teaspoon (2 g) black pepper**
- 6 **ounces (170 g) chopped ham**
- 1 **cup (285 g) full-fat Greek yogurt**
- 1 **cup (100 g) grated Parmesan cheese**
- 1 **teaspoon (5 g) yellow mustard**
- **Handful fresh parsley, minced**
- 1 **scallion, minced**

INSTRUCTIONS:

Melt the butter in a skillet over medium heat. Add the riced cauliflower, season with the sea salt and black pepper, and sauté until soft, about 5 minutes. Stir in the remaining ingredients until everything is well combined and heated through, about 5 minutes.

SERVES 2
PREP TIME: 5 MINUTES
COOKING TIME: 10 MINUTES

CALORIES: 612
CARBS: 24
PROTEIN: 48
FAT: 34

SEARED CHICKEN WITH PESTO AND TOMATOES

Keep staples such as prepared pesto sauce in your fridge for when you need some flavor and you need it fast. We love searing chicken and veggies and smothering it with pesto and Parmesan—get ready for your taste buds to love it too!

- 2 tablespoons (30 g) butter
- 2 (6-ounce/170 g) boneless, skinless chicken breasts
- 1 teaspoon (5 g) sea salt
- ½ teaspoon (1 g) black pepper
- ½ teaspoon (0.7 g) garlic powder
- 2 cups (400 g) cherry tomatoes
- ½ cup (120 g) pesto
- ½ cup (50 g) grated Parmesan cheese
- Lemon wedges, for squeezing
- Handful fresh parsley, minced, for garnish
- Minced fresh basil leaves, for garnish

INSTRUCTIONS:

Melt the butter in a skillet over medium heat. Add the chicken breasts and season with the sea salt, black pepper, and garlic powder. Scatter the cherry tomatoes around the chicken. Cover the skillet and sear the chicken until the internal temperature reaches 165°F (75°C), about 5 minutes per side.

Reduce the heat to low, smother the chicken with the pesto, and sprinkle the chicken and tomatoes with the Parmesan cheese. Cover the skillet again until the cheese is melted, about 1 minute. Remove from the heat and garnish with lemon juice, parsley, and basil.

SERVES 2
PREP TIME: 5 MINUTES
COOKING TIME: 15 MINUTES

CALORIES: 569
CARBS: 9
PROTEIN: 43
FAT: 41

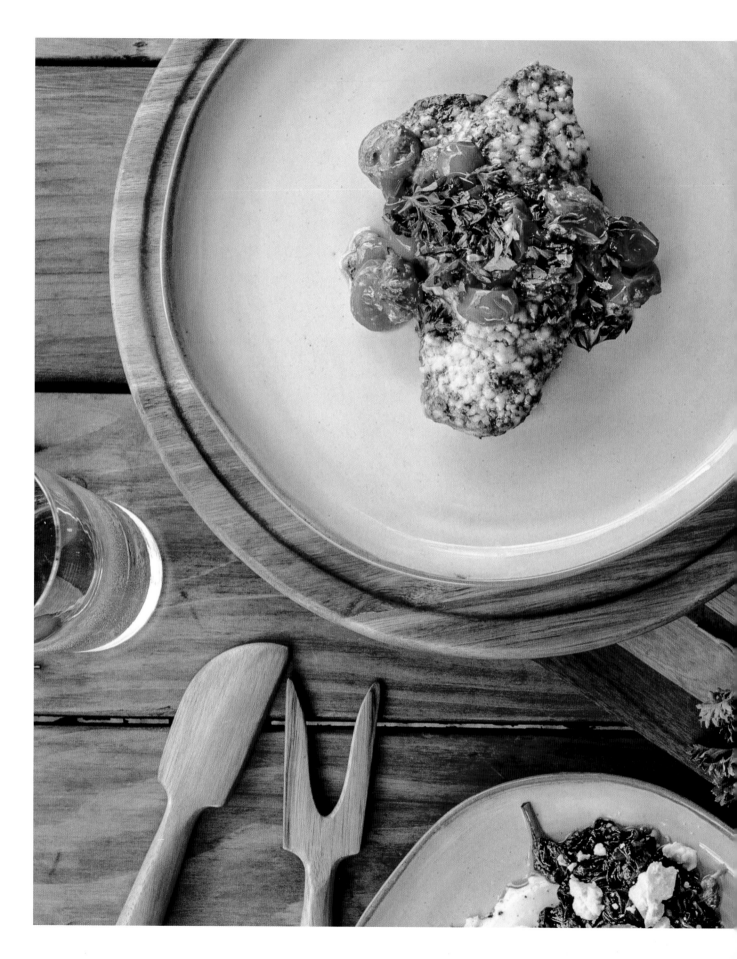

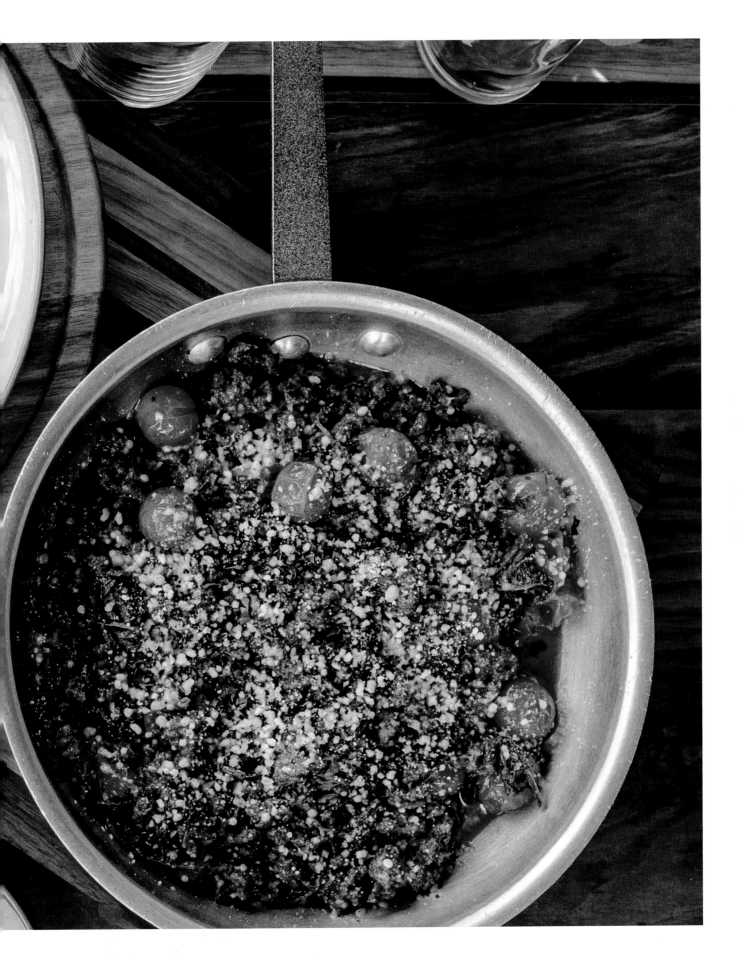

ITALIAN BEEF SKILLET

We keep our freezer stocked with high-quality ground beef so we can make quick meals such as this Italian beef skillet with tasty flavors from pesto, Parmesan, and parsley. This recipe takes only 20 minutes, so set your table and get your appetite ready!

- **2 tablespoons (30 g) butter**
- **1 pound (454 g) ground beef**
- **1 teaspoon (5 g) sea salt**
- **½ teaspoon (0.7 g) garlic powder**
- **2 cups (400 g) cherry tomatoes**
- **4 cups (120 g) baby spinach**
- **½ cup (120 g) pesto**
- **½ cup (50 g) grated Parmesan cheese**
- **Handful fresh parsley, minced, for garnish**
- **Minced fresh basil leaves, for garnish**

INSTRUCTIONS:

Melt the butter in a skillet over medium heat. Add the ground beef, season with the sea salt and garlic powder, and cook, stirring to break up the meat, 5–7 minutes. When the beef is about halfway browned, add the cherry tomatoes and allow them to burst open.

Drain off the excess fat, reduce the heat to low, and add the baby spinach. Sauté until the spinach is wilted, 2–3 minutes. Stir in the pesto and Parmesan cheese and cover the skillet until the cheese is melted, about 1 minute. Top with the parsley and basil.

SERVES 4

PREP TIME: 5 MINUTES

COOKING TIME: 15 MINUTES

CALORIES: 512

CARBS: 7

PROTEIN: 38

FAT: 36

BAKED EGGS

This meal is perfect for a crowd, as it's packed with protein and healthy fats and is made in one skillet so you can spend more time with your loved ones. Serve this alongside a salad of leafy greens and a dressing of olive oil, balsamic vinegar, and sea salt. Add some extra avocado or high-quality mayonnaise to amp up the fats if you prefer.

- 2 tablespoons (30 g) butter
- 1 pound (454 g) ground beef
- 1 teaspoon (5 g) sea salt
- 1 teaspoon (1.25 g) garlic powder
- 1 cup (200 g) cherry tomatoes
- 6 large eggs
- 2 cups (228 g) shredded cheddar cheese
- Minced fresh parsley, for garnish
- Minced fresh basil leaves, for garnish

INSTRUCTIONS:

Preheat the oven to 400°F (200°C).

Melt the butter in an ovenproof skillet over medium heat. Add the ground beef, season with the sea salt and garlic powder, and cook, stirring to break up the meat, 5–7 minutes. When the beef is about halfway browned, add the cherry tomatoes and allow them to burst open.

Drain off the excess fat from the skillet. Crack the eggs into the skillet on top of the beef and sprinkle with the cheese.

Bake until the eggs are done to your liking and the cheese is melted, 10–15 minutes. Garnish with parsley and basil.

SERVES 6
PREP TIME: 10 MINUTES
COOKING TIME: 20 MINUTES

CALORIES: 401
CARBS: 2
PROTEIN: 30
FAT: 29

TUNA AND AVOCADO SALAD

This is a fast meal requiring no cooking, so it's perfect for any meal of the day. Add some fresh or dried herbs to enhance the flavor even more!

- 2 tablespoons (30 mL) extra-virgin olive oil
- ½ teaspoon (2.5 g) sea salt
- Grated zest and juice of ½ fresh lime
- ½ scallion, minced
- 1 (5-ounce/142 g) can tuna packed in water, drained
- 1 medium (150 g) avocado, peeled, pitted, and chopped
- ½ cup (75 g) sliced red bell pepper
- ½ cup (60 g) sliced cucumber

INSTRUCTIONS:

Whisk together the olive oil, sea salt, lime zest and juice, and scallion in a bowl. Gently toss in the tuna, avocado, bell pepper, and cucumber until coated in the vinaigrette.

SERVES 1

PREP TIME: 5 MINUTES

CALORIES: 656

CARBS: 7

PROTEIN: 28

FAT: 50

CHIPOTLE CHICKEN BURGERS

Aim to use dark-meat ground chicken in this recipe to keep the fat content high and the flavor amazing! Avocado and sour cream make these burgers extra satisfying, so dig in and enjoy!

- 12 ounces (342 g) ground chicken
- 1 teaspoon (5 g) sea salt
- 1 teaspoon (2 g) black pepper
- 1 tablespoon (7 g) chipotle powder
- 2 tablespoons (30 g) butter
- 2 (1-ounce/28 g) slices pepper Jack cheese
- 4 cups (160 g) mixed salad greens
- 1 medium (150 g) avocado, peeled, pitted, and sliced
- ¼ cup (60 g) full-fat sour cream

INSTRUCTIONS:

Combine the ground chicken, sea salt, black pepper, and chipotle powder in a bowl and mix with your hands. Form 2 equal patties.

Melt the butter in a cast-iron skillet over medium heat. Cook the chicken patties until cooked through, about 4 minutes per side. Place a slice of cheese on each patty and let it melt.

Serve the patties on a bed of mixed greens, topped with avocado and sour cream.

SERVES 2
PREP TIME: 10 MINUTES
COOKING TIME: 10 MINUTES

CALORIES: 563
CARBS: 8
PROTEIN: 41
FAT: 36

BUTTER SALMON AND GREEN BEANS

Fresh and easy, this meal is a reminder that eating great doesn't have to be complicated or take a long time. All you need is a skillet and a few staple ingredients.

- 4 **tablespoons (60 g) butter, divided**
- 12 **ounces (100 g) French green beans**
- 1 **teaspoon (5 g) sea salt**
- ½ **teaspoon (1 g) black pepper**
- 1 **teaspoon (1.25 g) garlic powder**
- 12 **ounces (342 g) wild-caught, skin-on salmon**
- 4 **cups (160 g) mixed salad greens**
- ½ **cup (58 g) chopped hazelnuts**

INSTRUCTIONS:

Melt 2 tablespoons of the butter in a cast-iron skillet over medium heat. Add the green beans, season with the sea salt, black pepper, and garlic powder, and sauté for 5 minutes. Push the green beans to the side of the skillet and add the salmon, skin side up. Sear until cooked through, about 1–2 minutes (or 3–4 minutes if it's a thick cut).

Serve the salmon and green beans on a bed of mixed greens, topped with the remaining 2 tablespoons butter and the chopped hazelnuts.

SERVES 2
PREP TIME: 5 MINUTES
COOKING TIME: 10 MINUTES

CALORIES: 558
CARBS: 7
PROTEIN: 34
FAT: 45

BAKED PESTO SALMON

Keep staples such as high-quality mayonnaise and pesto in your fridge so that you can make dishes like baked pesto salmon whenever the mood strikes!

¼ cup (60 g) mayonnaise

½ cup (120 g) pesto

4 cups (160 g) baby spinach

12 ounces (342 g) wild-caught, skin-on salmon

1 teaspoon (5 g) sea salt

½ teaspoon (1 g) black pepper

½ cup (58 g) chopped walnuts

INSTRUCTIONS:

Preheat the oven to 400°F (200°C).

Mix the mayonnaise and pesto in a small bowl.

Arrange the baby spinach in a baking dish and place the salmon on top, skin side down. Spread the mayonnaise-pesto mixture over the salmon and bake until the salmon is pale pink and flaky, 15–20 minutes. Season with the sea salt and black pepper and top with the chopped walnuts.

SERVES 2

PREP TIME: 5 MINUTES

COOKING TIME: 20 MINUTES

CALORIES: 410

CARBS: 6

PROTEIN: 23

FAT: 34

FRIED EGGS TO THE RESCUE

Sometimes you need a very fast meal, and when you do, eggs come to the rescue! Fry them up with sea salt and black pepper and serve with tangy feta cheese and creamy avocado.

- 2 tablespoons (30 g) butter
- 3 garlic cloves, minced
- 4 cups (160 g) baby spinach
- 4 large eggs
- 1 teaspoon (5 g) sea salt
- ½ teaspoon (1 g) black pepper
- 2 ounces (56 g) feta cheese, crumbled
- 1 medium (150 g) avocado, peeled, pitted, and sliced

INSTRUCTIONS:

Melt the butter in a cast-iron skillet over medium heat. Add the garlic and cook until golden and fragrant, about 1 minute. Add the baby spinach and sauté until wilted, about 1 minute. Push the spinach and garlic to the side to make room for the eggs. Crack the eggs into the skillet, season with the sea salt and black pepper, and cook until the whites are cooked through, 2–3 minutes. Serve topped with feta cheese and sliced avocado.

SERVES 2

PREP TIME: 5 MINUTES

COOKING TIME: 5 MINUTES

CALORIES: 493

CARBS: 9

PROTEIN: 23

FAT: 40

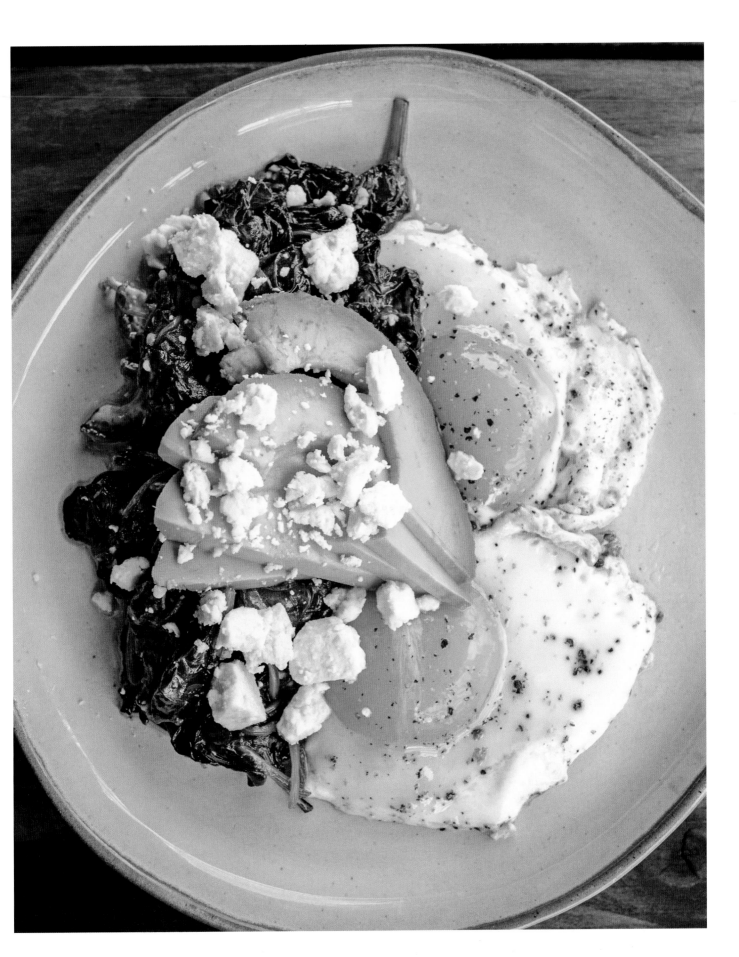

ACKNOWLEDGMENTS

Tremendous thanks to the dream team who supported this project. Sarah Steffens (SavorAndFancy.com) slaved away in the grocery store and in the kitchen to help dream up, test, and refine the recipes. Sheila Curry Oakes came through under pressure with another magnificent editing job on her second *Two Meals a Day* book project. The spectacular recipe photos from Natalie Brenner Photography LLC were a joyous team effort from the best talent Portland, Oregon, has to offer: Chef Kiara of Kitchen Killa, Chef Ceejay of PDX Munch Time, and Kiana of Muse Cheesecakes for styling and plating. Layout and design by Toni Tajima.

Celeste Fine, John Maas, and Anna Petkovich of Park & Fine Literary and Media and Suzanne O'Neill of Grand Central Publishing believed in the *Two Meals a Day* project and lifestyle movement from the very beginning and have made the authors' dream into a reality.

The highest acknowledgment is extended to you, our readers, for having the courage and dedication to take responsibility for your health. We sincerely appreciate your interest and look forward to connecting with you further at TwoMealsADayBook.com, SavorAndFancy.com, MarksDailyApple.com, and BradKearns.com.

RESOURCES AND SUGGESTED READING

Books

The Art and Science of Low Carbohydrate Performance, by Jeff Volek, PhD, RD, and Stephen D. Phinney, MD, PhD

Body by Science, by Doug McGuff, MD

The Bordeaux Kitchen, by Tania Teschke

Boundless, by Ben Greenfield

Boundless Cookbook, by Ben Greenfield

The Carnivore Code, by Paul Saladino, MD

The Carnivore Code Cookbook, by Paul Saladino, MD

Carnivore Cooking for Cool Dudes, by Brad Kearns, Brian McAndrew, and William Shewfelt

The Carnivore Diet, by Shawn Baker, MD

The Case Against Sugar, by Gary Taubes

The Circadian Code, by Satchin Panda, PhD

Death by Food Pyramid, by Denise Minger

Deep Nutrition, by Catherine Shanahan, MD

The Diabetes Code, by Jason Fung, MD

Eat to Live, by Joel Fuhrman, MD

Fast Food Nation, by Eric Schlosser

Fat Chance, by Robert H. Lustig, MD

Fat for Fuel, by Joseph Mercola, MD

The Fatburn Fix, by Catherine Shanahan, MD

Food Politics, by Marion Nestle

Good Calories, Bad Calories, by Gary Taubes

Grain Brain, by David Perlmutter, MD

Keto Cooking for Cool Dudes, by Brad Kearns and Brian McAndrew

Keto for Women, by Leanne Vogel

The Keto Reset Diet, by Mark Sisson with Brad Kearns

The Keto Reset Diet Cookbook, by Mark Sisson with Lindsay Taylor, PhD

The Keto Reset Instant Pot Cookbook, by Mark Sisson with Lindsay Taylor, PhD, and Layla McGowan

Lights Out, by T. S. Wiley with Bent Formby, PhD

The Longevity Paradox, by Steven R. Gundry, MD

Lore of Nutrition, by Tim Noakes and Marika Sboros

The New Evolution Diet, by Arthur De Vany, PhD

The Obesity Code, by Jason Fung, MD

The Overfat Pandemic, by Dr. Philip Maffetone

The Paleo Diet, by Loren Cordain, PhD

Paleo Happy Hour, by Kelly Milton

The P:E Diet, by Ted Naiman, MD, and William Shewfelt

Perfect Health Diet, by Paul Jaminet, PhD, and Shou-Ching Jaminet, PhD

The Plant Paradox, by Steven R. Gundry, MD

The Primal Blueprint, by Mark Sisson

The Real Meal Revolution, by Tim Noakes, MD, Jonno Proudfoot, and Sally-Ann Creed

The South Asian Health Solution, by Ronesh Sinha, MD

Wheat Belly, by William Davis, MD

Why We Get Fat, by Gary Taubes

You: The Owner's Manual, by Michael F. Roizen, MD, and Mehmet C. Oz, MD

Websites

TwoMealsADayBook.com (contains hyperlinks for all the books, websites, videos, and shopping resources mentioned here; a comprehensive list of research links, including videos, interviews, health journalism, news reports, and scholarly articles; plus bonus content and ebook downloads)

AncestralSupplements.com/about-us (Brian "Liver King" Johnson, ancestral living tips and inspiration)

AndreObradovic.com (Australian life and endurance training coach)

BenGreenfieldFitness.com (biohacker, podcast host, elite adventure athlete, and bestselling author of *Boundless*)

BradKearns.com (*Two Meals a Day* coauthor, podcast host, and elite athlete)

CarnivoreMD.com (Dr. Paul Saladino, carnivore leader and author of *The Carnivore Code*)

CulturalHealthSolutions.com (Dr. Ronesh Sinha, author of *The South Asian Health Solution*)

DeniseMinger.com (blogger, author, and conventional wisdom skeptic)

DietDoctor.com (Dr. Jason Fung, insulin, obesity, and diabetes expert)

DoctorJKrauseND.com (Dr. Jannine Krause, naturopathic doctor, acupuncturist, and podcast host)

DoctorOz.com (Dr. Mehmet Oz, bestselling author and TV personality)

DrCate.com (Dr. Catherine Shanahan, NBA diet consultant and bestselling author of *Deep Nutrition*)

DrDaphne.com (Dr. Daphne Miller, integrative physician and advocate of nature-based healing)

DrFuhrman.com (Dr. Joel Fuhrman, bestselling author of *Eat to Live*)

DrGundry.com (Dr. Steven Gundry, bestselling author of *The Plant Paradox*)

DrJoeDispenza.com (neuroscientist, author, and peak-performance expert)

DrPerlmutter.com (Dr. David Perlmutter, bestselling author of *Grain Brain*)

DrRagnar.com (Dr. Tommy Ragnar Wood, ancestral health expert and pediatrics researcher)

DrWeil.com (Dr. Andrew Weil, bestselling author and natural-medicine expert)

ElleRuss.com (podcast host and bestselling author of *The Paleo Thyroid Solution*)

EvolutionaryAnthropology.duke.edu/people/Herman-Pontzer (Dr. Herman Pontzer, author of *Burn*)

FacultativeCarnivore.com (Amber O'Hearn, carnivore-diet advocate)

FoodPolitics.com (Marion Nestle, bestselling author, researcher, and antipropaganda advocate)

GaryTaubes.com (science journalist and bestselling author of *Good Calories, Bad Calories*, *Why We Get Fat*, and *The Case Against Sugar*)

HealthfulPursuit.com (Leanne Vogel, podcast host and bestselling author of *The Keto Diet*)

Instagram.com/TheUsefulDish (Lindsay Taylor, social psychologist and coauthor of *The Keto Reset Diet Cookbook* and *Keto Passport*)

KetoGains.com (Luis Villasenor, bodybuilder and founder of ketogenic-diet and coaching service)

MarksDailyApple.com (my number-one-ranked ancestral-living blog, home of the Primal Blueprint lifestyle; contains extensive library of articles, success stories, and free ebook downloads)

MarksDailyApple.com/keto/keto-results/Brian-McAndrew (Brian McAndrew's body-transformation story)

MarksDailyApple.com/ancestral-resting-positions (my research with Matt Wallden)

MichaelPollan.com (health journalist and bestselling author of *The Omnivore's Dilemma*)

MyCircadianClock.org (Dr. Satchin Panda's time-restricted feeding app and research)

PaulJaminet.com (astrophysicist, ancestral diet expert, and coauthor of *Perfect Health Diet*)

PerfectHealthDiet.com (Shou-Ching Jaminet, molecular biologist, cancer researcher, and coauthor of *Perfect Health Diet*)

PeterAttiaMD.com (surgeon, podcast host, longevity expert, biohacker, self-experimenter, and extreme endurance athlete)

Shawn-Baker.com (orthopedic surgeon, carnivore-diet leader, world-record-setting masters rowing athlete, and founder of MeatRx.com)

ThePaleoDiet.com (Dr. Loren Cordain, health and exercise science professor, Paleo researcher, and bestselling author of *The Paleo Diet*)

WestonAPrice.org (Weston A. Price Foundation, a leading resource for the global study of the diet and health habits of indigenous peoples)

WheatBelly.com (Dr. William Davis, cardiologist and bestselling author of *Wheat Belly*)

YouTube Videos

Use these search terms:

Brad Kearns—A Day In The Life

Brad Kearns—Chest Freezer Cold Water Therapy

Brad Kearns—Dynamic Stretching Routine to Start Your Day

Brad Kearns—How to Do a Sprint Workout the Right Way

Brad Kearns—Morning Routine

Brad Kearns—Preworkout Dynamic Stretching Routine

Brad Kearns—Running Form: Correct Technique and Tips to Avoid Injury

Brad Kearns—Running Technique Drills: Beginners

Brad Kearns—Running Technique Drills: Advanced

B.rad Podcast—Dr. Cate Shanahan: How to Become Cancer Proof

B.rad Podcast—The Ultimate Mark Sisson Interview

Fillet-Oh!-Fish [fish farm industry exposé]

Hatha Yoga for Beginners

The Great Dance: A Hunter's Story [San bush people persistence hunt]

Jeanne Calment Interview [world's oldest human, lived 122 years]

Joe Rogan—Mark Sisson Interviews #1 (2017) and #2 (2021)

Mark Sisson—Amazing Keto and Fasting Facts

Mark Sisson—Archetypal Rest Postures

Mark Sisson—BASS (Bigass Steak Salad)

Mark Sisson—A Day in the Life

Mark Sisson—Keto Roundtable: Metabolic Flexibility and the Human "Closed Loop" System

Mark Sisson—Micro Workouts How-To and Benefits

Mark Sisson—Health Theory [why the keto diet will change your life]

Mark Sisson—Primal Essential Movements

Mark Sisson—Sprinting Workout

Mark Sisson—What Is Intermittent Fasting?

Pilates at Home for Beginners

Restorative Yoga for Beginners

Tai Chi for Beginners

Yoga Sun Salutations

Internet Shopping Resources

AncestralSupplements.com (100 percent grass-fed animal organ supplements)

Askinosie.com (artisan bean-to-bar dark chocolate)

BarAndCocoa.com (Distributor of artisan bean-to-bar dark chocolate)

ButcherBox.com (sustainable animal foods; home delivery club)

ChiliTechnology.com (chiliPAD mattress cooler)

CocoaRunners.com (UK-based distributor of artisan bean-to-bar dark chocolate)

DrinkLMNT.com (sugar-free electrolyte drink mix)

Evolution-Athletic.com (resistance bands)

GrasslandBeef.com (US Wellness Meats 100 percent grass fed beef, with plentiful organ meats)

IrisTech.co (screen color-temperature-optimizing software)

JustGetFlux.com (screen color-temperature-optimizing software)

LillieBelleFarms.com (dark chocolate)

LoneMountainWagyu.com (100 percent purebred, grass-fed Wagyu beef)

MeatRx.com (carnivore diet community and educational programming)

NZCordz.com (StretchCordz and other resistance-training bands)

PerformBetter.com (Mini Bands)

RAOptics.com (fashionable blue light–blocking eyewear)

ThriveMarket.com (healthful organic foods with online discount)

VariDesk.com (stand-up desks and creative office furniture)

VitalChoice.com (wild-caught seafood with home delivery)

WildIdeaBuffalo.com (grass-fed, naturally raised buffalo from the Great Plains)

X3Bar.com (X3 Bar home strength-training device with resistance straps)

INDEX

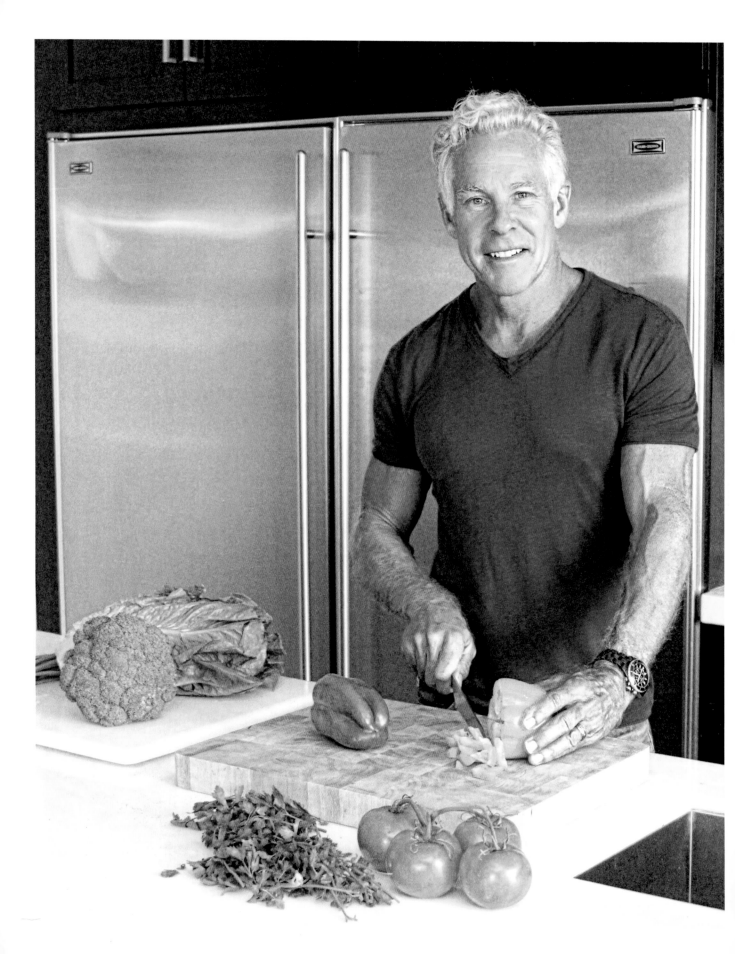

ABOUT THE AUTHORS

MARK SISSON is widely regarded as one of the forefathers of the ancestral health movement. A former world-class athlete in the marathon and Ironman Triathlon, he presides over a wide-ranging Primal enterprise, featuring the Primal Kitchen line of healthy condiments, the Primal Health Coach Institute, a line of premium performance and nutritional supplements, and numerous books and online educational courses. He publishes daily tips and inspiration at MarksDailyApple.com, the top-ranked blog in its category for the past fifteen years. Mark lives in Miami Beach, Florida, with his wife, Carrie, where he standup-paddles the inland waterways, plays ultimate Frisbee against hotshots half his age, and enjoys his new role as a grandfather.

BRAD KEARNS is Mark Sisson's longtime co-author, host of the *B.rad* podcast, and elite masters athlete. He broke the Guinness World Record in Speedgolf at age 53, reached the #1 USA-ranking for age 55–59 high jumpers in 2020, and is a former US national champion and #3 world-ranked professional triathlete. Brad lives in Lake Tahoe, Nevada, with his wife, Elizabeth, and enjoys a daily cold plunge in the lake year-round.

SARAH STEFFENS loves to create delicious meals that leave your body feeling nourished, strong, and happy. When she's not cooking up tasty food for her loved ones and clients, she's soaking up nature in Northern California, reading a good memoir, or geeking out over an old movie shot in wide angle. Catch more of her recipes on Instagram @sarahsteffens_personalchef.

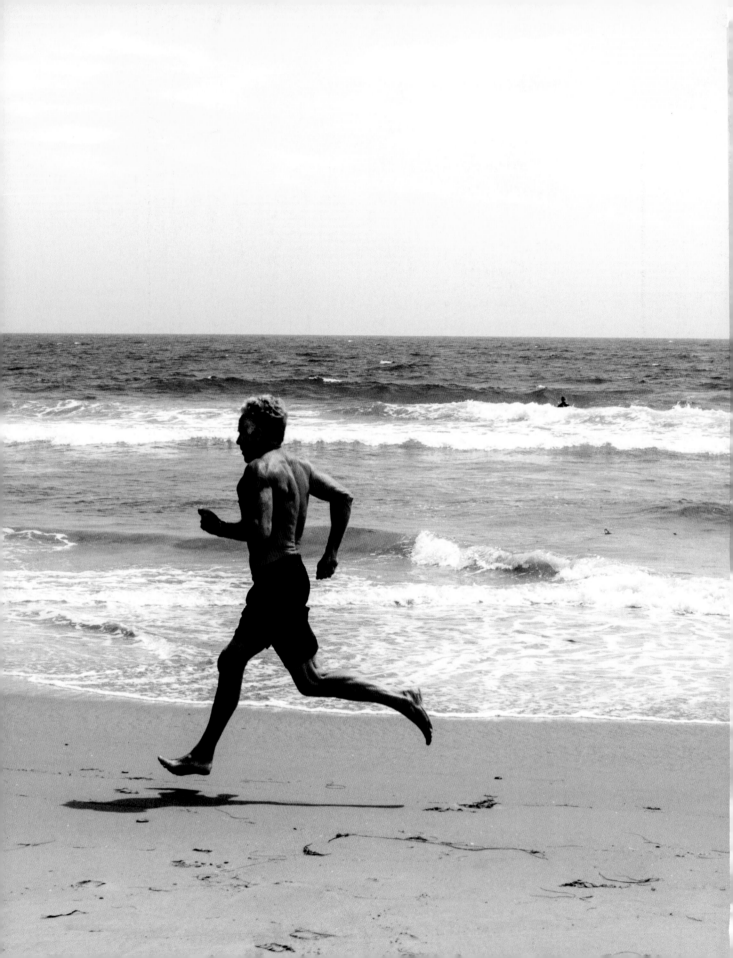